BODY ON FIRE

How Inflammation Triggers Chronic Illness
and the Tools We Have to Fight It

Monica Aggarwal, MD
Jyothi Rao, MD

Healthy Living Publications
Summertown, Tennessee

Library of Congress Cataloging-in-Publication Data

Names: Aggarwal, Monica, author. | Rao, Jyothi, author.
Title: Body on fire : how inflammation triggers chronic illness and the
  tools we have to fight it / Monica Aggarwal, Jyothi Rao.
Identifiers: LCCN 2020022093 (print) | LCCN 2020022094 (ebook) | ISBN
  9781570673924 (paperback) | ISBN 9781570678288 (epub)
Subjects: LCSH: Inflammation—Prevention. | Chronic diseases—Prevention. |
  Self-care, Health. | Nutrition.
Classification: LCC RB131 .A38 2020 (print) | LCC RB131 (ebook) | DDC
  616/.0473—dc23
LC record available at https://lccn.loc.gov/2020022093
LC ebook record available at https://lccn.loc.gov/2020022094

DEDICATION

I dedicate this book to Rob.
You are my light.
Knowing you are with me
is my greatest strength and power.

MONICA AGGARWAL, MD

I dedicate this book to my late father,
Ramachandra Rao,
for the incredible role model and influence
he was and still is in my life,
and to my late maternal grandfather,
Dhruva Rao,
who inspired me to heal others.

JYOTHI RAO, MD

CONTENTS

v

FOREWORD

Finding New Tools to Heal the Whole Body

W e live in a world that relies heavily on conventional medicine and, especially, pharmaceutical drugs to manage disease conditions. For acute and critical problems these approaches have tremendous value, but they are less useful in cases of chronic illness, many of which result from unhealthy lifestyle choices. I have been researching alternative healing practices for more than 40 years. After completing my training in conventional medicine, I traveled the world, living with and acquiring knowledge from people of many different cultures. Most of the healing systems I have studied emphasize the role of food choices and sleep, along with natural remedies, mind/body techniques, and spiritual practices, to maintain and restore health. Combining some of these ideas and methods with conventional medicine has been the foundation of the integrative medicine that I teach and practice.

Body on Fire is an engaging book that recounts the parallel journeys of two skilled physicians, Dr. Monica Aggarwal and Dr. Jyothi Rao, who were motivated to find new tools that would enable them to heal the whole body, not just treat symptoms. I first met Dr. Aggarwal, an energetic and accomplished cardiologist, in 2005. She had a thriving practice, with a commitment to provide the best care for her patients, but she was already aware of the limitations of pharmaceuticals and curious about alternative therapies. When she was diagnosed with rheumatoid arthritis in 2011, her search for other ways to treat began in earnest. Dr. Aggarwal offers a frank discussion of her debilitating disease and her path to healing. I am impressed by her transformation and evolution as a physician and how she has learned to incorporate her discoveries into caring for her patients. The positive outcome she experienced is an inspiring testament to the power of choice and control we have in matters of health.

Dr. Jyothi Rao is a dedicated internist who has long held the belief that healing the body involves much more than pills. More and more providers are struggling with the same frustration with conventional medicine that she felt. It led her to pursue acupuncture and functional medicine to help her patients. I admire her relentless effort to create an integrative internal medicine practice that is demonstrating how nonpharmacologic modalities can change lives.

The book these two doctors have written is a useful resource for anyone interested in attaining better health. The authors explain how both lifestyle choices and environmental triggers can cause breakdowns in various body systems, and they offer prescriptions with detailed practical tips to correct them. Anyone can make use of this advice to have lasting benefits with only positive side effects. Drs. Aggarwal and Rao draw on available scientific data to support their points and are not afraid to say when data are lacking.

We know that our health is not predetermined by genes alone. It is our day-to-day choices of how we live, environmental influences, stressors, and how we handle them that determine health outcomes. The experience of illness is not the same for everyone with the same diagnosis. Treatment must be individualized—there is no one size that fits all. And the impact of lifestyle changes will also differ from person to person. But I believe the information and tools that Drs. Aggarwal and Rao present in these pages are applicable to all of us and can serve as a guide to achieving optimum health.

ANDREW WEIL, MD

INTRODUCTION

Body on Fire

We have one body. We have one life. Everything we do to it from our birth to our old age has an impact. When we are young, we believe we are invincible. We feel we can stress our bodies and they will endure. And they will at the beginning. We keep doing the things we do because we often don't feel the impact until years later. The body is prepared for stress. We have stress hormones and systems in place that allow us to deal with stress. Our senses become activated and we are more keenly aware of our surroundings. Our immune system is revved up and we are able to deal with insults. But at some point, with more continuous stress, our demand outweighs our resources. Our bodies have only so much reserve, and ultimately, our bodies become imbalanced. These stresses come from many external sources, such as excess sunlight, pollution, lack of sleep, and social and job stress, as well as lack of activity. Stress also comes from the foods we ingest such as processed foods, meat, and dairy.

When the body becomes imbalanced, it becomes irritated and inflamed. We call that "body on fire." The body becomes so revved up that the insides become unhappy. The immune system goes into overdrive and switches from a controlled system into a wild, overcharged system that can start hurting itself. It can start attacking its own organs. This inflammation over time ultimately leads to illness. Inflammation manifests differently in everyone. Some people have stomach complaints: constipation, abdominal pain, and diarrhea. Some people experience excessive fatigue, weight gain, and depression. Others develop autoimmune disease, such as multiple sclerosis, rheumatoid arthritis, and inflammatory bowel disease. Still others develop cancer and heart disease. Initially, when we don't feel right, we consult our physicians, who see little wrong in the baseline lab results. In further testing, certain markers of inflammation might be elevated but not always at the beginning. These normal test results can leave us feeling unsatisfied and give a false sense of security. Ultimately, we end up ignoring signs or they are too nonspecific for doctors to pinpoint the diagnosis. Then we develop sickness and are surprised how it happened. We, the authors, know because it has happened to us.

We are all affected in some way or another. It always takes a toll. It is for this reason that we, Dr. Aggarwal (a cardiologist) and Dr. Rao (an internist), have decided to write this book. We have been sick. We know what it feels like to be blindsided by illness, yet the signs were there all along. We just weren't looking. As physicians, we started to look for answers first in our pills. When the pills left us with nasty side effects and incomplete healing, we started on a journey to understand why the body gets sick and what we can do to heal it—truly heal it. Over the years, we have learned together that there is so much we can do to put our bodies back in balance. There are so many options for treatments, beyond our pills, to heal our bodies and decrease our inflammation. We have written this book to educate you, to offer you hope for options for healing and to empower you with the knowledge and tools to identify your fires and extinguish them.

Healing is not a simple task . . . but it is a worthwhile one. As physicians, we stand by the medicines that we prescribe, but we offer here additional prescriptions that don't come in pill form. These are prescriptions that complement our medications and sometimes, if we are lucky, allow us to stop taking our pills. It happened for us, and it happens for so many of our patients. Here, in these chapters, we give you a comprehensive and detailed study and present as much data as is available on these matters. The reality, however, is that much of the data out there is not the desired randomized control trial. There are few studies that will compare diet with pills because of the worry of withholding therapy and because there is a significant lack of funding. Often, studies are funded by pharmaceutical companies. Pharmaceutical companies want trials, because if there are positive associations between illness and the medication they prescribe, we physicians will prescribe that medication and pharmaceutical companies will make more money. The problem is that the prescriptions in this book aren't pills. Companies have no incentives to offer solutions that don't include drugs.

Therefore, we present as much data as we could find and as many anecdotes as we could, and you can make your own judgments. These tools can and should be used with a standard medical treatment plan. Consider how little you have to lose by trying these prescriptions and how much you could possibly gain. We are not prescribing dangerous changes. You will suffer no medication side effects if you follow our advice. What do you have to lose by trying? These prescriptions changed our lives by extinguishing our fires. We hope they will change yours too. We want you to be empowered to change, to heal, to balance. Come with us on this journey. Welcome to the new and healthier you!

As you read through this book, we ask you to consider how you feel. See table 1 where we have listed questions for you to ask yourself. If you answer "yes" to any of these questions, we hope you will take the time to read this book.

TABLE 1: HOW DO I FEEL?

ENERGY

- ☑ Do I feel as if I don't have the energy to do the things I want to do daily?
- ☑ Do I feel tired when I wake up in the morning?
- ☑ Do I feel as if I need a nap during the day, such as right after lunch?
- ☑ Am I in pain when I wake up, or do I feel pain throughout the day?

LIFESTYLE

- ☑ Is it hard to find the energy to exercise?
- ☑ Am I frustrated with my weight?
- ☑ Do I feel like I am taking too many pills?
- ☑ Do I feel like I need more sleep?

FOOD

- ☑ How do I feel after eating my food? Do I get tired? Does my pain get worse?
- ☑ Are my meals healthy? What does that look like? Does my food come in a frozen box? Do I cook or mainly microwave?
- ☑ I really don't eat anything, but do I feel like I continue to gain weight?
- ☑ Do I feel constipated? Do I only go to the bathroom every few days?
- ☑ Do I crave sweets all of the time?

MIND

- ☑ I've had bad habits my whole life. Can I still change?
- ☑ Do I feel anxious all of the time?
- ☑ Do I have difficulty with my memory? Do I forget where I park my car?
- ☑ Do I have trouble falling asleep at night because my mind is always moving?

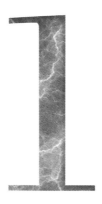

A Juggling Act

BALANCE, INTERNAL STABILITY, AND HOMEOSTASIS

*Homeostasis: The tendency of the body to create
internal stability and equilibrium, despite stressors.
It is the body's need to have balance.*

omeostasis is the concept that our bodies strive to stay in balance without any excesses or depletion of resources, and it is the foundation for staying healthy. No over- or under-stimulation. Balance. It is what our bodies desire, and it is vital to keeping our bodies healthy, stable, calm, and free of illness.

Our bodies have many adaptive mechanisms for maintaining homeostasis. In times of stress and trauma, we activate various hormones to bring our systems back into balance. Day-to-day activities trigger these adaptive devices. But often, we expose ourselves to too much stimulation, excessive stresses, and overuse. Our bodies then become depleted of resources and cannot maintain homeostasis. We lose our balance—and without balance, our bodies suffer and we develop illness.

Stress comes from many places. Stress comes from pressures at home and work. It comes from what we put into our bodies, such as recreational drugs or medicinal ones. It comes from the food we put

1

into our bodies. It comes from lack of sleep and overstimulation. In this modern era, we have so many external stimuli. We are continually receiving information through our computers and phones. We have the internet to answer our every question. We receive information through our smartphones that notify us of every weather change, of important news bulletins, and of every email and text from people who want to communicate with us. We are constantly moving. Our society is always "on." We go to bed with the glow of tablets at our bedsides and wake to the buzzing of text messages and social media notifications. The stimulation is immeasurable. Each of these stresses impacts our bodies. These stresses disrupt the internal homeostasis. Our bodies have to use an abundance of resources to keep in balance again. But with time, those resources are lost and we become sick. This overuse leads to the onset of illness. (See Consider 1.)

CONSIDER 1

THE STRESS OF ALWAYS BEING CONNECTED

☑ How many times do you look at your phone when you are having a conversation with someone? At dinner? When you first wake up in the morning?

☑ Do you have audio notifications for all of your social media? Do you consider turning these off?

☑ How often do you check your email? How many times per hour? Can we just make a point to check them once every hour or every two hours instead of every time we hear the notification bell?

☑ Consider keeping your phone away from your bed, and plan a time after which you don't look at your phone. Maybe one to two hours prior to bedtime will be electronics free. If you use your phone as an alarm, get a different alarm.

We have many resources in our treasure chest. Those resources are our fuel and help us balance our bodies when they are being depleted by stress. Resources are in our foods, such as amino acids, omega-3 fatty acids, phytonutrients, and spices. Other resources come from nourishing good gut bacteria and stimulating detox and anti-inflammation pathways with sleep, sunlight, meditation, and exercise—and much more. (See Figure 1 on the next page.)

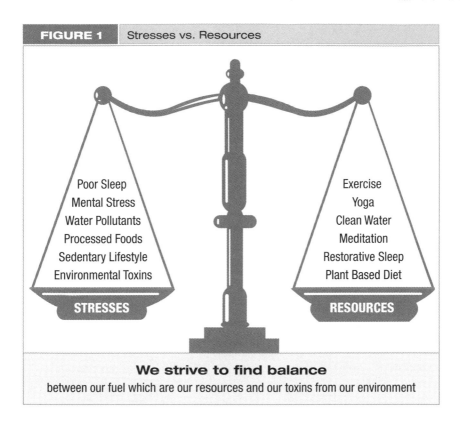

FIGURE 1 | Stresses vs. Resources

Poor Sleep
Mental Stress
Water Pollutants
Processed Foods
Sedentary Lifestyle
Environmental Toxins

STRESSES

Exercise
Yoga
Clean Water
Meditation
Restorative Sleep
Plant Based Diet

RESOURCES

We strive to find balance
between our fuel which are our resources and our toxins from our environment

Over the centuries, there has been a surge in the prevalence of many illnesses, such as obesity, heart disease, cancer, and autoimmune disease. We are seeing more heart attacks in younger people; more lung cancers in nonsmokers; and more lupus, rheumatoid arthritis, and inflammatory bowel disease. One could argue that we see more of these diseases now because people are living longer and getting more age-related diseases. But we have to consider, as well, that in the current day, there are many more toxins and stresses our bodies are exposed to, triggering more illnesses.

Today in medicine we have become quite advanced and have learned to treat many of these illnesses. We have learned to treat cancers with chemotherapy and radiation. We have learned to treat high blood pressure with pills. We have learned to treat clogged heart arteries with pills and then stents. If the heart becomes weak, we have learned how to put in mechanical hearts and do heart transplants. If the joints go bad from excess weight, we replace the joints.

We have become a society that focuses on fixing messes instead of preventing them. We install new joints before we discuss weight loss and building muscle. We perform gastric bypass (weight-loss) surgery before we educate people on what they can eat to lower their risk of obesity. We prescribe cholesterol-lowering agents and blood pressure medicines before we teach people about sodium and cholesterol, saturated fats, and trans fat. Our insurance covers antidepressants before it covers psychotherapy. We do not focus on root causes of illness, such as stress and inflammation-induced imbalances, but only the end result. With all of the advancements in health and technology, are we any better? Are we healthier?

As patients, we, too, look for magic pills to cure whatever ails us. We want pills that cause us to lose weight. We ask our doctors to prescribe pills to give us energy and ease pain in our joints. We look for pills that clear up our skin and treat our allergic reactions. We want to eat whatever we want and then take a pill to treat the resulting high blood pressure, high cholesterol, and heart disease.

But there are no magic pills. Every pill has a side effect, a cross-reaction, a potential adverse reaction. If you have taken medications before, you know this to be true. So let us try to move away from the lure of magic pills and instead implement lifestyle interventions that will give us the best chance to become healthy. Let us be empowered and go on this journey together! See Consider 2.

CONSIDER 2

BROKEN PILL PROMISES

- ✓ Every pill has a side effect.
- ✓ There are no magic pills.
- ✓ Would you rather take a pill for every ailment or make an intervention that has a lasting effect?

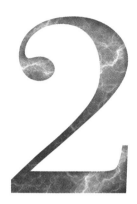

How My Daughter Saved Me

Dr. Monica Aggarwal's Story

When I was little, I used to think that I didn't bleed. I was never injured and rarely even received a cut. When my son was born, I remember laughing at myself because of my surprise that when he fell, he would bleed. For some crazy reason, I think we all believe when we are little that we are invincible. I carried that feeling of invincibility into my 30s. I was a powerhouse. I worked hard and long hours, then came home and crashed, only to wake up and do it again the next day.

I felt I had it all. It is a tricky thing being a career woman, though. We spend our lives studying to reach the top of our game, but then that goal often coincides with the years when we want to have children. I had three children in five years. I poured the same intensity from my training years into my children. I nursed them all. I made fresh meals daily, baked their birthday cupcakes, and knit their Halloween costumes. I was exhausted. It was a hard life, but I felt that it was a burden I had to accept in order to have it all.

After my third child was born, life changed for me. I recall the time so vividly. I went back to work eight weeks after the baby came. I remember the utter exhaustion of sleeping for three hours, going to work, then running home to nurse, cook meals, and start the routine all over again. Every night my husband would drag me out of one of our children's bedrooms so I could fall asleep in my own bed, until the next cry woke me up. I was haggard. I felt I had to sacrifice myself temporarily to have it all. One morning, four months after my third child was born, I woke up to the baby's cry and I couldn't move my right shoulder. It was red and hot. I ignored it and figured it was a trauma I couldn't remember. Three days later, my left fourth finger was red and hot. I started having trouble buttoning the kids' clothes. A day later, I felt like glass shards were piercing the bottoms of my feet.

I still ignored the pain. I started taking the elevator at work because my feet hurt too badly to climb the stairs and I couldn't bend my knees. After about a week, I knew that something was really wrong. I recall the day vividly, almost as if it was a dream. The alarm went off at 5:30 a.m. I remember feeling exhausted in my bones. I could barely get out of bed. I hobbled down the stairs to let the dog out, but my feet were worse than ever. The glass kept cutting my feet. I made it downstairs, but I could barely open the door to let the dog out. Then the baby cried. I started to run up the stairs on impulse, so as not to let the other children wake with the noise, but I couldn't get there. I couldn't run. Every bone in my body burned. I couldn't climb the stairs to reach her. I can still taste the salt in my mouth from my tears as I crawled up the stairs. I remember reaching her crib but not being able to lift her out. It was then, as I lay on the floor crying so that my husband had to pick up the baby and give her to me, that I realized I was in real trouble.

Two weeks later, I had a diagnosis of severe rheumatoid arthritis (RA). My rheumatologist looked at my inflammatory markers and told me that my prognosis would be a severe, debilitating course if I didn't begin advanced therapy immediately. After my first meeting, I was fairly sure that I would no longer be able to practice cardiology. All of the pictures from medical school of advanced RA came flooding back. The baby was now five months old and I was nursing. My rheumatologist told me to stop nursing as soon as possible, because he was very concerned about the destructive signs that my lab markers portended and about how symptomatic I was. He wanted me on drugs within one week.

So I followed his advice. I stopped nursing my baby. I cried every moment of those seven days. Every time I heard the baby cry, I had to walk away. My breasts were engorged and painful, yet I could not feed her. I still want to cry as I write this because of the deep sorrow I felt at those moments. I felt my choice was taken away from me; I had to give up something that was so dear to me. But every patient learns quickly that you have few choices. As patients, we have to rely so much on our physicians and suspend our own disbelief.

As I started losing my hair and my daily nausea became more severe, I felt more and more bitter and lost. I started to blame my daughter. I thought that if I hadn't had a third child, none of this would have happened. After a few months of being on the medications, though, I started to feel better. I became better adjusted to the drugs and had fewer side effects. It was around that time that I started coping with my disease, but I still hadn't released the anger. I still blamed my little girl for my disease. One day, about six months after beginning my treatment, I met a woman who would soon become a dear friend. She was a holistic nutrition consultant and was interested in educating my patients about diet. I was immediately skeptical, and she offered to do my nutrition profile. It was then that I started considering the effects of the foods we eat on inflammation in our bodies.

It is commonly thought that people develop illness after their bodies receive multiple insults. The first insult is often genetic, and then environmental triggers add to the initial insult. For instance, a person may be genetically predisposed to heart disease (the genetic insult) and have high LDL (bad cholesterol) and low HDL (good) cholesterol levels. Then she adds a diet rich in saturated fats and hydrogenated oils, plus a sedentary lifestyle and smoking (the environmental insults), and we have a young woman with premature heart disease. Similarly, with cancers, there is likely a genetic component, then we suffer some sort of environmental insult that creates stress (oxidative stress), which then triggers the abnormal cells to arise.

Those environmental insults or triggers can be different things to different people—lack of sleep, cigarettes, excessive sun, saturated fats, gluten, or dairy. Understanding what causes their inflammation is the key. **We believe that when you change your diet, remove stressors, and make anti-inflammatory choices, you can decrease inflammation.**

It takes time to learn our own bodies' sensitivities. Dairy and other animal products are often the source of inflammation. I was already vegetarian, so I started with dairy elimination. I cried when I gave up my pizza. Like most Americans, I also worried about not getting enough calcium and protein in my diet. It took me a lot of self-teaching to understand that so much of our calcium and protein comes from the beans and greens we are eating.

It took me four years to admit to others that I had an illness. I always felt that if I said it out loud, people would judge me or think I was less adequate as a physician, as a mother, and as a person. Now I realize it is because I have an illness that I understand and connect with my patients better. I can relate to their reluctance to take a medication. I feel their fear as if it were my own. I feel their helplessness and anger as the fire in my own heart. I also know now that, at the end of the day, we are all affected. Then, it is about learning to avoid environmental triggers and nurturing our bodies with a plant-based diet, low in oils and refined sugars, and undergoing lifestyle changes, such as increased sleep and more vigorous activity.

It has taken me a long time to embrace my disease. I have learned that it is not illness that defines us but, rather, how we respond to it that makes us who we are. A person like me who was so controlled and rigid falls hard when illness hits. I blamed my poor daughter for being the cause of my illness. I was angry for a long time. But now I feel healthier than ever before. My cholesterol is super low. My inflammatory markers are nonexistent, and I take no medications. I am strong. Two years after my diagnosis, I came off all of my medications. Soon after that, I did my first triathlon. Six years later, I remain off *all* medications. I feel great. I have learned to take time for myself. I have learned to laugh more and not worry so much about being late or about climbing a ladder. I thank my body every day for what it has to give me, and I forgive it for what it cannot. In some ways, the crazy thing is that getting sick was the best thing that happened to me. I have my girl to thank for bringing me back from a world in which I was drowning. I realize now that my daughter didn't make me sick; she saved me.

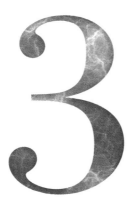

Learning the Meaning of MD

Dr. Jyothi Rao's Story

M y grandfather was a true physician, not only because of his knowledge or clinical acumen, but also because he tended to his patients where they lived and worked. He made house calls, even in the middle of the night, for treatments ranging from minor surgery to counseling—he was always ready with a warm smile or a hand to hold. He helped those in need, those without any money, those who were scared about pain and illness. In his rural community in India, he was a hero and was beloved . . . and I wanted to be just like him.

Visiting patients in the home is not practical, but it does offer advantages. It provides the ability to see people holistically, in their life roles, and identify the stressors they encounter every day. It gives insights into their struggles with socioeconomic class, family dynamics, and living conditions. My grandfather was able to identify the root cause of an ailment with much more ease since he knew, really knew, his patients. He made a difference in their quality of life. Ever since I can remember, I wanted to do exactly that. I wanted to help guide people to thrive. I wanted to bring some comfort back into their lives.

I went to medical school yearning for knowledge and eager for experience in treating illness. I pursued positions in which I would work with those who were dedicated, knowledgeable, and devoted to their patients. My residency was in a tertiary care (specialized treatment) medical center where I saw a wide variety of ailments and worked alongside great and caring physicians who were leaders in their fields. I finished my residency empowered with the feeling that I now possessed the knowledge to follow in the path of my grandfather.

However, starting in private practice in New York, I was overwhelmed when I realized how little we as physicians could do to actually heal. Sure, we could diagnose illness and treat symptoms, but what about addressing the cause of the problem? Why put someone on a vigilance drug for daytime sleepiness when we should be looking for a solution to their sleep issues? We did extensive workups on many patients who had concerning symptoms, only to find everything was "normal." So, is it normal to have achiness all over? Is it normal to not have a bowel movement for five days? A city that takes pride in never sleeping provides an environment rich with stress-related symptoms, such as insomnia, irritable bowel syndrome (IBS), migraines, palpitations, and many more.

Why is weight gain such a big problem? Where is the joy and vitality in everyone? There was not enough time to counsel or delve deep into sources of stress, which I felt was the root of 75 to 80 percent of what I see in internal medicine. What happened to bringing comfort back into our patients' lives? After all of my study and hard work and aspirations to help people, all I had in my toolbox were bandages. I wrote prescriptions and briefly discussed exercise and diet. I was a fireman, putting out fires that had already started and doing nothing to prevent future fires from igniting.

It was at this point that I decided to train in acupuncture, so I could offer more wellness tools to my patients. I learned about the concept of energy movement and began looking at the root cause of illness. Using acupuncture in my practice gave me a new paradigm shift. It was not only a tool for common symptoms such as back pain, migraines, acid reflux, and many other everyday illnesses I was treating, but I also heard from patients that they felt more energetic, they slept better, and their mood improved. As I learned about creating balance, I felt empowered once again. I could teach my patients about elementary prevention, which is keeping systems in balance so illness doesn't have a chance to strike. I was finally on the path to integrative, functional medicine.

No longer do we have to feel that we are destined by our genes. We have the tools to impact the ways in which our genes manifest themselves. Functional medicine allows me to delve into genetic variations, the impact of oxidative stress, nutrient imbalance, and how different environmental toxins break down our bodies, according to varying socioeconomic conditions and climate exposure. These differences change the ways our bodies respond to stress and create oxidative stress and inflammatory changes. These pathways of inflammation lead to our symptoms and to different disease states.

It was in my postgraduate years that I learned how to keep people well. It is my goal to educate people about the multitude of various stressors in our lives, ranging from the environmental (poor air and water quality, extreme climate changes, poor food quality with pesticides, and GMO and processed foods), to the chemical (toxins in water and medication side effects) to the mental (feeling out of control).

I continue to strive to find tools that allow me to practice medicine the way my grandfather did—holistically. I continue to search for knowledge that will empower my patients. Aging is an inevitable part of life. I want to teach my patients not to fear it but to embrace aging. We may not be as fast, our joints may feel creaky, and we may have more wrinkles on our faces. But we can be strong. We can be at peace and free of chronic illness. It is all about balance.

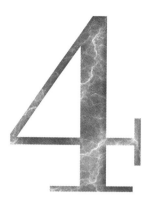

Breaking Down

When balance is disrupted, stress and inflammation are created—
the role of our central nervous system.

We now know that imbalance in our bodies can cause illness. Now, let's understand which factors create imbalance in the first place.

Imbalance is prompted by stress and can be brought on by an injury, anxiety, toxins we ingest, lack of activity, and many more triggers. The powerful effect of stress on your body is the most important concept that we will relay to you, because if you recognize how stress works, you can then start the healing process. The term "stress" was coined in the 1950s by Hans Seyle, MD, a pioneer in the field of endocrinology.[1] Some consider him the first researcher to examine the biological impacts of stress and the connections between the mind and body. He defined stress as a body's response to a demand for change. Stress can be emotional, mental, physical, chemical, or environmental. It can be a physical reality or created in our minds, but in either case it sets off a fixed reaction in our bodies. Seyle broke down stress into *eustress* and *distress*.

Eustress is good stress driven by positive anticipation, such as when we are expecting a child, starting a new job, or planning a vacation. It refers more to the way our body reacts to stress. It gives us good coping skills and makes our senses hyperacute. Distress, on the other hand, is negative stress and triggers inflammation and oxidative stress. Distress occurs when we suffer the loss of a child or spouse, termination of a job, or divorce. Both situations demand that the body change. (See figure 1 and Consider 1.)

CONSIDER 1

 Do you have more distress or eustress in your life?

Dr. Seyle was a pioneer because he saw the connection the mind has over the body. He formed our current thinking around general adaptation syndrome, the ways in which our bodies cope with stress. During times of changing environment or a perceived threat, our acute stress response is adaptive and allows us to cope and respond appropriately to survive the stress. An acute stress response in healthy individuals is a good thing. It is a normal process, and it is protective.[1] In acute stress response, we see activation of the nervous system and the cardiovascular, endocrine, and immune systems. The goal of the stress response is to release resources for the body to make energy for immediate use. The body also starts to allocate these resources to specific organs and shuts down resources to other organs to help conserve energy.

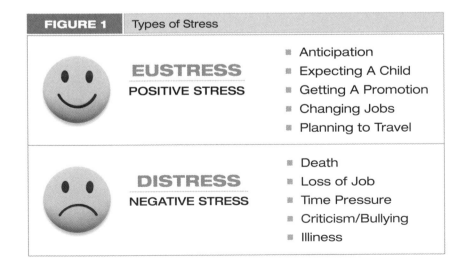

FIGURE 1	Types of Stress
EUSTRESS POSITIVE STRESS	▪ Anticipation ▪ Expecting A Child ▪ Getting A Promotion ▪ Changing Jobs ▪ Planning to Travel
DISTRESS NEGATIVE STRESS	▪ Death ▪ Loss of Job ▪ Time Pressure ▪ Criticism/Bullying ▪ Illness

When our senses perceive a threat, the *autonomic nervous system* is triggered. The two major components of the autonomic nervous system are referred to as the sympathetic and the parasympathetic nervous systems. These systems are regulated by neurotransmitters, or chemical signals, which communicate to the nervous system to set off a chain of responses. They work in balance to affect many systems of the body, such as the heart, eyes, stomach, and genitals. The sympathetic nervous system (SNS) is also called our fight-or-flight system. The SNS triggers the release of neurotransmitters, such as epinephrine and norepinephrine, which then signal the cardiovascular system to increase blood pressure and heart rate. The heart pumps faster and gets blood to all essential organs more quickly, so the body is ready for whatever comes its way. It also suppresses gut motility and the urge to urinate so that we aren't hungry when we are running and do not have the urge to urinate or defecate. The SNS also increases blood flow to our skeletal muscles and our brain. Our eyes dilate so we can see better in the dark. All of our senses become keener, we are more alert, and our muscles can endure. Simultaneously, the parasympathetic (PNS), our rest and digestive system, is suppressed. This system is responsible for lowering blood pressure, lowering heart rate, and improving gut motility. When there is an acute stressor, activities not essential for immediate survival, such as digestion, growth, and reproduction, are suspended.[2]

Another major pathway that becomes activated when stress is perceived comes when a signal in our brain triggers the release of cortisol (from the adrenal gland, the stress response center). Cortisol has two main jobs. The first is to help make energy. It is responsible for breaking down fat (lipolysis) and making sugar from storage sources (glycogenolysis). It also mobilizes fat from the periphery to the center to prepare it for use.[3] (See figure 2 on the next page.)

Its second role is to regulate the immune system. Without overwhelming ourselves here with how immunology works, the role of cortisol is to balance inflammation with anti-inflammation. Our acute stress response allows for an increase in white cells—the infection fighters (macrophages and natural killer cells) that go into tissues, such as our skin or other organs, and act as protection against those cells most likely to suffer damage during an insult. Our immune system recruits chemicals in our blood to help fight against new trauma, infection, or injury.

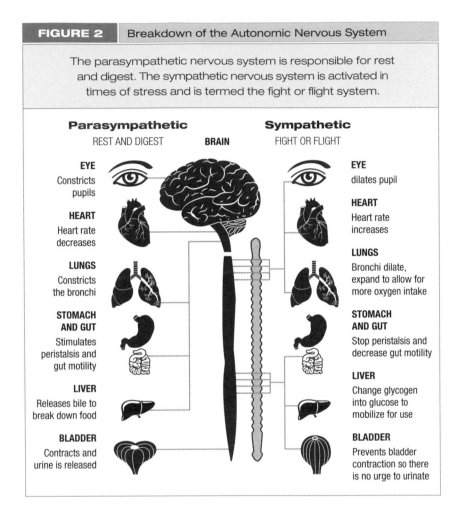

FIGURE 2   Breakdown of the Autonomic Nervous System

The parasympathetic nervous system is responsible for rest and digest. The sympathetic nervous system is activated in times of stress and is termed the fight or flight system.

Parasympathetic
REST AND DIGEST

BRAIN

Sympathetic
FIGHT OR FLIGHT

EYE
Constricts pupils

HEART
Heart rate decreases

LUNGS
Constricts the bronchi

STOMACH AND GUT
Stimulates peristalsis and gut motility

LIVER
Releases bile to break down food

BLADDER
Contracts and urine is released

EYE
dilates pupil

HEART
Heart rate increases

LUNGS
Bronchi dilate, expand to allow for more oxygen intake

STOMACH AND GUT
Stop peristalsis and decrease gut motility

LIVER
Change glycogen into glucose to mobilize for use

BLADDER
Prevents bladder contraction so there is no urge to urinate

One of the benefits of cortisol in acute stress is that it suppresses our pain response. When we are being chased, we cannot worry about the pain in our muscles or minor injuries. This is a protective benefit. It allows us to run despite injury. Cortisol is also known to be a catabolic hormone, which means it breaks down parts of our body, such as our muscle and bone, to provide nutrients to help us weather a stressful time. Again, when we are running from a tiger, we need all of the energy we can muster to save our lives. Cortisol is responsible for keeping us moving in times of stress. (See figure 3.)

People often ask whether cortisol is good or bad. Cortisol levels are a measure of stress. They are cyclic in the body. When we first

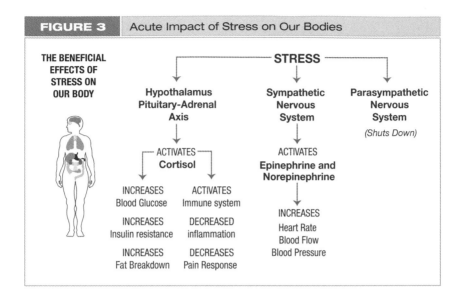

FIGURE 3 | Acute Impact of Stress on Our Bodies

THE BENEFICIAL EFFECTS OF STRESS ON OUR BODY

STRESS

Hypothalamus Pituitary-Adrenal Axis

Sympathetic Nervous System

Parasympathetic Nervous System
(Shuts Down)

ACTIVATES
Cortisol

ACTIVATES
Epinephrine and Norepinephrine

INCREASES
Blood Glucose

ACTIVATES
Immune system

INCREASES
Insulin resistance

DECREASED
inflammation

INCREASES
Heart Rate
Blood Flow
Blood Pressure

INCREASES
Fat Breakdown

DECREASES
Pain Response

wake up in the morning, our cortisol levels are at their highest. It is believed that those high amounts are needed then to mobilize our bodies for the day.[3] A way to think about cortisol is that it gives us our "get-up-and-go" and allows us to be prepared for whatever the day holds. In a healthy state, these levels gradually decrease during the day.

However, in times of external stress, cortisol levels shift, and they become elevated at times when they would normally decline. This is necessary to activate our fight-or-flight response, to mobilize energy, and to allow us to meet the demands of a stressful day. Imagine a mother watching her child in a park and she witnesses him falling from the monkey bars. She sees her child on the ground, crying in pain and unable to walk. Her alarm phase kicks in, and she is mobilized to get her child help. We can see then that the stress response is extremely important.

Chronic Stress Response

When is stress detrimental to our health? If stress becomes persistent, our cortisol levels become chronically high. With the case of the mother who watches her child fall from the playground equipment, she learns her child has a broken bone in his leg, and she must fully care for him for six weeks while he is in a cast. This results in persistent high cortisol levels with constant activation of her fight-or-

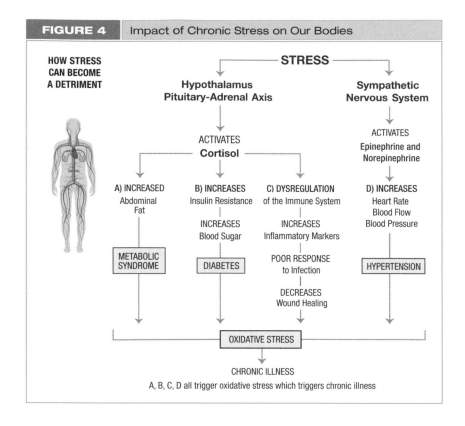

FIGURE 4 | Impact of Chronic Stress on Our Bodies

flight response. Her heart rate and blood pressure are continuously elevated. Her muscles are broken down, and fat is pulled from the periphery. (See figure 4.)

People with high cortisol levels often have trouble with excessive abdominal weight (apple shape). Their sugar levels are also chronically elevated. The immune system becomes overactivated and this can lead to suppression of key immune functions. This suppression can lead to increased risk for infections. Have you noticed, in times of stress that you are more prone to getting a cold? If the stress is ongoing, exhaustion sets in, preventing us from adjusting to the stressful situation. This is where the stress response takes the form of burnout, overtraining, or exhaustion. In the case of our mother from the playground, she has poor sleep, poor support, and poor nutrition, which can leave her burned out after six weeks of constantly caring for her child.

In times of burnout, there is significant imbalance in the immune response. We see more inflammatory markers, decreased wound healing, and poorer response to infection.[2] Further, it has been shown that with chronic stress there is overactivation of the hormonal systems and subsequent formation of disease-causing free radicals. Free radicals are toxic to our cells. Their formation and injury to cells is called *oxidative stress*.[4] Inflammation and oxidative stress can then cause chronic fatigue, depression, and excessive weight gain. In addition, persistent elevation of cortisol can lead to insulin resistance, which can cause chronic disease states, such as diabetes and cardiovascular disease. Chronic stress can lead to higher levels of anxiety, increased depression, and insomnia. Other functions, such as cognition, memory, and reproduction, are also adversely affected.[4] (See Consider 2.)

CONSIDER 2

☑ Do you get sick more often when you are stressed?

☑ Is your memory worse when you are stressed?

Remember that cortisol is about the balance between inflammation and anti-inflammation. In chronic stress, that balance is disrupted, and even with high levels of cortisol, the body becomes resistant and the balance with anti-inflammation is lost.[5] This can cause a marked increase in inflammatory cells and can trigger an autoimmune disease in which the body actually starts attacking itself.[6]

Cortisol plays a role in aging as well. First, let's discuss how aging affects the body. Aging is defined as the process of growing old, and this involves every cell in our bodies. Chronologic age is the number of years we are alive, but a person's biological age may be different, depending on different insults to their systems. That is why we see so-called age-related illnesses at different ages in different people.

All cells in the body are continually dividing. It is a necessary function of life. All cells have genetic material (genes) in them that assign the cells their jobs. The genetic material defines who we are and how we think. Our genes are carried in our chromosomes. Chromosomes have caps on the ends called telomeres, whose job is to protect genetic material and promote chromosomal stability. Each time a cell divides, chromosomes are split, but the telomeres shorten because they cannot replicate with each splitting. Telomere shortening has been correlated with the aging of cells. Ultimately, without telomeres, our cells stop dividing. Without cell division, the body cannot repair and is prone to illness and dysfunction. This expedites biologic aging. Chronic stress is associated with shorter telomere length, which can then cause cells to stop dividing, and, ultimately, is associated with increasing biological age. In other words, chronic stress may be associated with premature aging and the onset of age-related illness. This is an area of great interest right now.[7]

Consider what age-related illnesses can do to us. With age, lung capacity is reduced, digestive enzymes in our guts decrease, brain size can shrink, and the cushions between the disks in our spines can grow smaller, causing us to actually lose height. Functionally, as we age, cognitive function diminishes. Vision weakens, as well as other senses, such as smell and hearing. The fat-to-muscle ratio grows, causing metabolism to slow down. Collagen in the skin dwindles and the skin thins. Our immune systems become weakened, and sleep disturbances increase. Stress can exaggerate the rate of our physical decline. In general, as we age, the risk of chronic disease grows. We desperately need tools to help lower our stress responses if we want to slow aging of our cells. (See Consider 3.)

CONSIDER 3

✓ What stresses do you have in your life that are triggering your inflammation?

- Consider where you multitask in your life and whether there are ways to reduce this.
- Do you stand and eat your dinners?
- Do you do other things while eating—use your cell phone, read the newspaper?
- Do you take on more work or activities than you can handle?

With constant stimulus, are we at our most efficient? Consider a cheetah who runs to pursue its prey. After it catches the prey, it spends time resting and recharging. That rest-and-recharge time is the counterbalance to the fight-or-flight response and is essential for healing the body. It is during this time that the parasympathetic nervous system is activated and blood pressure and heart rate slow down. Our hunger response returns, and digestion returns to normal. Our pain response comes back, and we can spend time healing our wounds. Our cortisol levels drop as well, so we stop breaking down muscle and fat; we can again build our fat and muscle stores. We return to having a normal immune response to insults.

Now, in our current day-to-day lives—with constant motion, work stress, and overstimulation from our electronic devices and poor nutrition that causes body aches, lack of activity, and lack of sleep—our bodies are under constant stress. Imagine if your phone battery showed a 7 percent charge rate; you would panic. Your primary mission would be to find a charger. Think of your body that way. It needs a battery charger, and if you don't have time to rest and recharge, you are prone to an inflammatory state that cannot recover from injury. You cannot heal. This is the state within which most of us lead our lives. When you read Dr. A's personal story, you will see that she certainly was overstressed. And with that condition came illness, as it often does. Most of us don't see how stress and overstimulation affect us until we have suffered real injury.

YOUR PRESCRIPTION

Some stressors are good and protective. Too much stress can be toxic and inflammatory. Stress can be

- mental
- physical
- environmental

Learn to identify your eustress from your distress.

1. Think about saying "no" to more requests during the week to allow time to relax and recover on weekends.

2. Schedule fewer activities for yourself and your family to allow for more personal time.

3. Learn to outsource where able.

4. While eating, chew slowly. Eat small meals more frequently. Don't multi-task while eating.

5. Don't check your email every five minutes. Concentrate on checking only once per hour.

6. Turn off computers, electronic tablets, and phones one to two hours before bedtime to allow the mind to calm down.

See Figure 1: Eustress versus Distress (page 14)

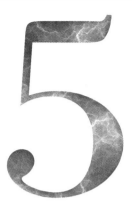

Chronic Illness
Is Born

CASE 1: Patient HB is a 39-year-old man who is a physical education teacher in a high school. He weighed 326 pounds. When he came to see Dr. A, his blood pressure was in the 190/70 mmHg range (very high). His LDL cholesterol was 160 gm/dL, and his triglycerides were 360 gm/dL. He showed signs of prediabetes. His EKG had already changed to show strain from the blood pressure. Dr. A put him on blood pressure medications and an intensive diet. She put him on an exercise plan. He lost 100 pounds. His blood pressure came into the 120 mmHg range. His LDL cholesterol dropped into the 130 gm/dL range, and his triglycerides came down into the 150 gm/dL range (normal). He felt like he could keep up with his students and was feeling better.

CASE 2: JS is a 45-year-old accountant who is morbidly obese with diabetes, hypertension, and atrial fibrillation (abnormal heart rhythm). He had sleep apnea (intermittently using a CPAP machine to keep his airways open so he could get enough oxygen at night). He was a former wrestler and wanted to get back to it. He came to see Dr. A for preoperative clearance to treat an injured toe. Dr. A put him on medication to control his heart rate and manage his blood pressure. She insisted on the patient's compliance with use of their CPAP machine. She put him on a plant-based, whole-grain diet. He was the perfect patient. He lost 65 pounds, came off of some of his blood pressure medications, and decreased medication for his blood sugar. His heart rates were better controlled, and he felt great. Dr. A sent him for foot surgery, and after the three-month healing of his toe, he started to wrestle again. He said he couldn't believe he was wrestling again. He didn't think he would ever get back to it.

How We Become at Risk for Illness

Many of the illnesses we see in our practices are due to a disruption in balance. In this chapter, we are going to explore what has happened to illness over the decades.

Heart disease, stroke, and cancer are the top killers of men and women around the world.[1] In America, we are seeing more lung cancer, breast cancer, pancreatic cancer, and colon cancer than ever before. We also see more Alzheimer's disease, more autoimmune disease, and more osteoarthritis than in years past. (Figure 1)

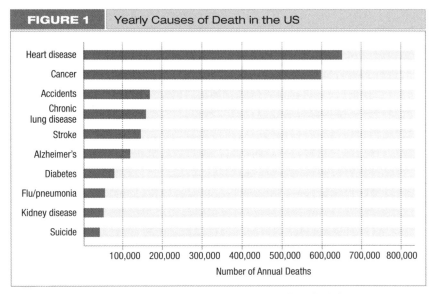

FIGURE 1 | Yearly Causes of Death in the US

Adapted from Deaths and Mortality, Centers for Disease Control. www.cdc.gov/nchs/fastats/deaths.htm

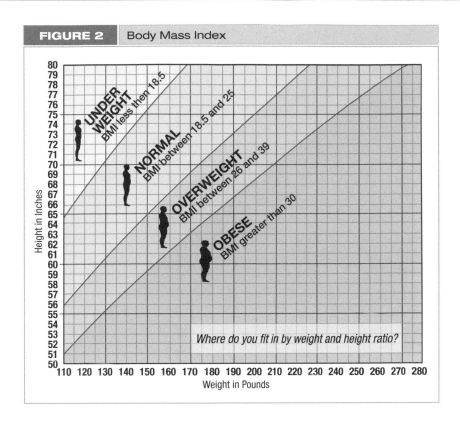

FIGURE 2 | Body Mass Index

Where do you fit in by weight and height ratio?

Height in Inches (vertical axis)
Weight in Pounds (horizontal axis)

UNDER WEIGHT — BMI less than 18.5
NORMAL — BMI between 18.5 and 25
OVERWEIGHT — BMI between 26 and 39
OBESE — BMI greater than 30

Over the decades, we have also seen individuals in our communities become more sedentary and gain more weight. Food preparation has shifted away from fresh food and cooking daily to ordering fast food and microwaving precooked or preprepared meals. Foods are filled with preservatives to increase their shelf life. Our jobs have become more sedentary. As a society, we work more and drive home in cars instead of walking. With these changes, we are fatter than ever before in history, with more than two of every three adults overweight or obese.[2] (See figure 2.) With that, the number of people with diabetes and prediabetes has reached 100 million people, and 10 percent of the US population is now diabetic.[3]

Let's talk for a moment about these illnesses in more detail.

Diabetes

aving diabetes puts us at significant risk for heart disease. We often find that people don't understand why diabetes is dangerous.

When we discuss diabetes in this book, we are primarily talking about type 2 diabetes, which is associated with obesity and insulin resistance. In order to understand diabetes, you have to understand the role of the pancreas. The pancreas is an organ in our bodies that makes the hormone insulin. The pancreas's job is to bring glucose into cells to build fat stores for later energy use. There are receptors on the pancreas for the insulin hormone. These receptors are like entry cards to get into cells. In the case of obesity or excess fat, there can be masking of the receptors on the cells, and the insulin hormone is not able to attach to these receptors. This is called *insulin resistance*. Without entry into cells, insulin isn't effective and doesn't get turned into fat. As a result, more sugar is floating around in the bloodstream. Some people might see that as positive and say, "If I can eat and not have it turn to fat, that's a good thing, right?"

Unfortunately, no. The problem is that floating sugars are extremely inflammatory, so as they circulate through the body, they irritate your blood vessels. They cause fissures in the blood vessels of the heart and cause scabs or plaque to form. The plaque migrates to the eyes and damages their small blood vessels, so people slowly lose their vision. As these scabs build in other blood vessels, they prevent blood from flowing to the various organs. Eventually, one of those blood vessels is completely blocked, and a part of the organ that the blood vessel supplies will die.

Studies show that weight loss can decrease blood sugars and correct diabetes.[4] Reducing simple carbohydrates and refined sugars will help reduce insulin resistance and diabetes. It seems, then, we have the ability to change the course of the disease, and with the reduction of diabetes, there will be a reduction of cardiovascular disease. (See Consider 1.)

CONSIDER 1

Consider what you are doing to your body to put yourself at risk for diabetes.

Heart Disease

 et's talk about heart disease a little more, beginning with how it develops. Cardiovascular disease, often referred to as coronary artery disease or heart disease, is the formation of plaque in the coronary arteries. These arteries sit on the surface of the heart and supply blood to the heart so the heart can pump blood to the rest of the body. We often talk about these coronary arteries as the plumbing for the heart pump. When there is plaque buildup in the pipes, blood can't effectively flow through them and the heart can't pump well. Then there would be limited blood flow to the brain and other essential organs, causing damage to those organs. So, keeping the coronary arteries in good health is key to overall health.

How do we get plaque in our pipes, though? The *endothelium* is the inner layer of cells in all blood vessels, including the pipes in the heart—the coronary arteries. The endothelium is responsible for dilating the blood vessels to accommodate changes in activity level. When we exert ourselves, our blood vessels widen to allow more blood to flow through them, so it can reach the organs that need it. When we develop risk factors for heart disease, such as high cholesterol, high blood pressure, or smoking, the endothelium of the blood vessels becomes damaged. This is called endothelial dysfunction, which is the beginning of atherosclerosis (also known as coronary artery disease or heart disease). When the endothelium is damaged, it becomes rigid and does not dilate easily.

This damaged endothelium becomes a site for more plaque being deposited. Then platelets (which form clots) come to the site because they see damage to the blood vessel and start repairing the lining. This process of endothelial dysfunction and subsequent platelet adhesion (clot formation) creates the beginning of an atheromatous plaque, plaque forming on the insides of our artery walls. Think of this plaque like a scab on the body when it's injured. But unlike the outer surfaces of our bodies, where it does not matter how big the scab is because space is infinite, in a blood vessel it matters a great deal. The larger the scab, the more blood flow is obstructed. Blood can't get where it needs to go. (See figure 3 on the next page.)

As we develop more risk factors or the risk factors we have progress, more plaque adheres to the scab, and it gets bigger and bigger. When the plaque closes off the blood vessel completely, a person has a heart attack. There are two types of heart attacks. One type is where a small plaque or scab sitting in a coronary artery suddenly and randomly ruptures (explodes) in a blood vessel, and a 30 percent blockage of a blood vessel becomes a 100 percent blockage. That creates an acute

FIGURE 3 | How Plaque Forms in Our Blood Vessels

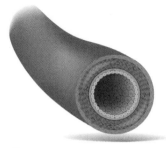

1 At birth, arteries are clear of obstructions

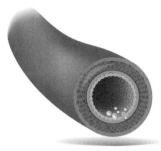

2 High blood pressure, smoking, high cholesterol can damage arteries walls

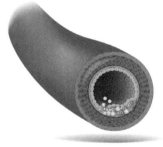

3 Scabs form, arteries grow rigid and do not dilate easily

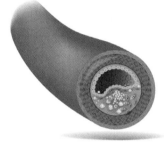

4 Plaque builds up over time with increased exposure to poor lifestyle habits

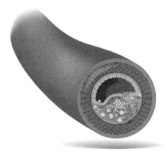

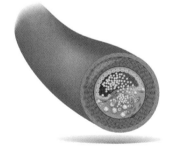

THE SPEED OF PLAQUE FORMATION

SLOW BUILD UP: Causes chest pain and possible less severe heart attack.

This is often less severe than the alternative because our bodies have had time to compensate for the decreased blood flow over time.

FAST BUILD UP: Plaque becomes irritated and ruptures, closing off the blood flow to vessel suddenly triggering acute heart attack.

Often, these heart attacks are dangerous and most serious because the body is unprepared.

heart attack and often results in death or heart failure. These are the heart attacks where patients are rushed urgently into our procedure labs and need to have a blood vessel opened quickly, usually with a stent.

The late actors James Gandolfini and Carrie Fisher died of this type of heart attack. We never know which of the scabs is going to rupture, but we do know that inflammation plays a role. Something irritates the cap of the scab, and it becomes susceptible to rupture, leading to subsequent blockage of the blood vessel. Interestingly, a plaque that has blocked 30 percent of a blood vessel is more likely to rupture and cause a major heart attack than one that has blocked 80 percent because the larger plaque has become calcified and hardened and is therefore less prone to rupture. Different imaging techniques help us understand which plaques are most prone to rupture, but the answer remains elusive. The best procedures we have are stress testing or taking X-rays of the heart arteries (to give something called a coronary calcium score) and measuring inflammatory markers that are specific to the heart. Highly sensitive C-reactive protein (hs-CRP) is a marker of inflammation, and this can often give us useful information that the heart is irritated.

The second type of heart attack occurs when blood flow demand and supply are mismatched. This happens when plaque builds up over time in the coronary arteries but doesn't always completely occlude the artery. It can also happen when there is another stressor, such as elevated blood pressure, infection, or anemia. The body needs the heart to pump blood to the other organs, but the coronary arteries are filled with plaque and the body can't get the heart to pump faster. As a result, people can develop chest pain and decreased blood flow to parts of the heart as well.

How can we decrease inflammation in the heart? We know that *statins* decrease the inflammatory marker, highly sensitive CRP, and can stabilize plaque, even when LDL cholesterol is not elevated. That is why so many of our cardiac patients are on statins. There are decades of data to show how effective statins are in reducing cardiovascular risk, and their benefits cannot be underestimated. There are also studies, however, supporting that many foods in our diet are inflammatory and cause the body to become irritated. Studies have shown that eating just one fatty meal can create endothelial dysfunction within four hours after the meal.[5] There are other studies that show how changing to a primarily plant-based diet will reduce inflammation and can decrease risk for cardiovascular disease.[6,7] Then there are other options besides pills to make us better! Yay! More on this on pages 53–72.

High Cholesterol

Cholesterol is an important substance for the body. It helps build the walls of our cells. It is the foundation of our sex hormones and important for formation of myelin sheaths, which are necessary for nerve conduction. When we have too much cholesterol, however, it finds other homes, such as in our heart arteries, head arteries, and legs. There are two main types of cholesterol: HDL (good cholesterol) that is responsible for removing cholesterol from the blood and taking it to the liver, and LDL (bad cholesterol) that puts it back into the blood vessel and helps to form plaque. When we are born, our LDL cholesterol levels are about 50 gm/dL. As our cholesterol levels go up with diet changes and other factors, we know we are more at risk for heart disease.

We often hear from our patients that their children "can afford to eat McDonald's food and fried chicken" because they are young. Is that really true? When we look at autopsies of children who died of unrelated causes, we find fatty streaks, signifying early plaque formation. Seventy-seven percent of men who fought in the Korean War had evidence of significant atherosclerosis. The average age of those men was 22 years.[8] Similar findings were seen in American men who fought in Vietnam.[9] This shows that the process starts at such a young age, and that what we put into our bodies at that young age matters. We can never afford to eat poorly. The bad foods that we eat as children put us at risk for heart disease and, as we will discuss later, for autoimmune disease, cancer, and other chronic illnesses as well. (See chapter 6 for details). The habits we create in children will last for a lifetime. It is so much easier to expose our children to healthy foods from the beginning so they will build a lifelong love of eating well.

Obesity and Hypertension

Before we talk about obesity, we need to define the terms. Obesity is often based on the body mass index (BMI), which is weight in kilograms divided by height (in meters) squared. There are many calculators available on the internet to aid in calculating your BMI. (See figure 2 on page 25.) Normal body mass indices are between 18.5 and 24.9 kg/m2. Being overweight is defined as having a body mass index between 25 kg/m2 and 29.9 kg/m2.[10] There are gradations of obesity, but for our purposes, obesity is defined as a body mass index of greater than 30 kg/m2. BMI is not a perfect assessment for obesity. BMI does not take into account thin people who have high fat percentages and central obesity (fat around the abdomen) or heavier people who have high muscle mass. We feel fat percentage and muscle mass are more informative than BMI. However, many of the national assessments are based on BMI. As noted earlier, as of 2009 over two-thirds of the population is considered overweight or obese.[11]

Being overweight and obese are associated with an increased risk of death.[12] In studies of overweight individuals above 50 years of age, there was nearly a 20 to 50 percent increased risk of dying.

What is it that our overweight and obese population is dying of? In one study, overweight men and women had a 52 percent and 62 percent risk, respectively, of death from cancer.[10] According to the Prospective Studies Collaboration analysis, when obese individuals were examined, a proportionately increased risk of heart disease, diabetes, cancer, and lung disease was found.[13] Cancers associated with increased weight, in particular, are liver cancer, kidney cancer, and breast, endometrial (uterine), prostate, and colon cancer. On the other hand, there are multitudes of studies to corroborate that the leaner we are, blood pressures decrease, sugars become more controlled, and we feel better.[14]

Obesity is strongly associated with high blood pressure (hypertension) and high cholesterol. Obese people typically eat more saturated fats and highly salted foods, which are felt to be significant causes of not only obesity but also of worsening blood pressure and high cholesterol. More than 100 million American adults, about 33 percent of the total adult population, have total cholesterol levels greater than 200 mg/dL (ideal is less than 200 mg/dL).[15] Of people with high cholesterol, about 67 percent of them are either overweight or obese. With the new American Heart Association hypertension guidelines, now almost 50 percent of Americans are considered hypertensive.[16]

Hypertension causes damage to the blood vessels, and high cholesterol boosts plaque formation. Both are directly linked to increased risk of heart disease. In the Framingham Study, obese people had more than twice the risk of heart disease compared to their leaner counterparts.[17] Obese individuals are more likely to have weakening of the heart or heart failure, as well as abnormal heart rhythms.

There is also a link between obesity and stroke, liver disease, and arthritis. The more weight we carry on our joints, the more traumas those joints suffer. Arthritis is one of the most costly morbidities associated with obesity. We have even linked skin changes, such as thickening of the skin (acanthosis nigricans), stretch marks, and increased hair production in women to obesity.

We weren't always so fat. We can all recall that when we were younger, people were smaller. When Dr. A was 20 years old, she weighed 120 pounds and wore a size four. Three babies and 15 years later, she now weighs a bit more than that, but she still wears a size four. Why is that? This is called *vanity sizing*. Retailers have gotten smarter. As people gained weight, they didn't fit into their usual sizes and needed bigger clothing. But people didn't want to buy larger sizes, so they didn't buy as many clothes. As a result, clothing manufacturers have adjusted their sizes to allow consumers to buy smaller-sized garments and feel skinnier. We heard a great story on *Hidden Brain*, Shankar Vedantam's show on National Public Radio, stating that a size six in 1970 would be comparable to a size two in 1996 and a size zero in 2012. Size zero! As we have gotten larger, we have changed our concept of what is normal. We are changing the sizes of our clothes to reflect that change, so we don't feel we are bigger. But we know that we are.

Many environmental factors contribute to obesity. Large portion sizes, high-sugar drinks, fast food, decreased physical activity, and watching more television are all linked to obesity. Television has been shown to directly influence our risk of obesity, and these trends are likely to follow into adulthood.[18]

Back in the old days, when people lived off the land, we were not an overweight population. We worked in the fields all day, picked our food for supper from the garden, and ate it while it was fresh. We ate more vegetables, fruits, and nuts. We lived off the land and only killed what we needed to feed our families. Nothing was wasted.

Over time, we have left our farms. We go to fast-food restaurants to get a quick meal as we drive to work. We sit for eight to ten hours per day and get up only to refill our sodas and eat meals. Often we are so busy that food is brought into meetings, so we don't have to break for a meal. We eat what is there and often much more than we need. We eat snacks and desserts because they are readily available. We then drive home and are usually too tired to exercise. We might eat a quick frozen dinner in front of the television and fall asleep. We snack until the late hours of the night. The sizes of our plates have gotten larger, so we eat more food. We drink less water and supplement with sodas and coffee to keep us awake because we are often tired. We eat pasta and simple sugars all day, so we have constant dips and plateaus in our energy levels. We then get a jolt of caffeine to keep us awake during the post-eating dips. Over time, we have become overweight and sedentary.

We have the ability to change this. Now that we have talked about the changes in chronic illness over time and the diseases our bodies are at risk for, we want to shift attention to the link between what we eat and how it changes the composition of our gut flora, which in turn activates abnormal body responses.

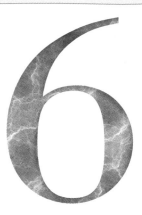

The House of Bugs

Learn about your gut

CASE: A 56-year-old woman with diabetes was recently admitted to the hospital for persistent, foul-smelling diarrhea. Recently, she had recurrent urinary tract infections and had been prescribed multiple courses of antibiotics. She was losing weight and had low energy. She was diagnosed with C. difficile colitis (an infectious inflammatory overgrowth in her gut) and was given more antibiotics to heal the infection of her gut. Despite multiple attempts at curing the infection, her diarrhea became intractable. She was given a fecal transplant, which is when the stool of a healthy family member is placed through a scope into the gut of the ill family member. Within weeks, the patient felt better; she was eating and no longer had diarrhea.

Learning about the gut is extremely important. It turns out that the gut has loads of bacteria in it. Those gut bugs are responsible for much of the immune system defense of our bodies and have a role in hormone and mood regulation. Those bugs also seem to have a role in decreasing inflammation and potentially a role in what illnesses we get. Before we go on, let's go over some definitions.

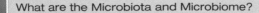

FIGURE 1	What are the Microbiota and Microbiome?

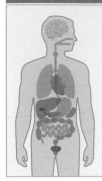

MICROBIOTA

Microorganisms (tiny bugs) in our bodies that are exposed to the outside surfaces. These include the gastro-intestinal organs (mouth to anus), skin, nose, ears and genitals.

MICROBIOME

Entire gene pool found in our bodies, so it includes the DNA (the brains) of every bug in our gut.

Microbiota is the term that refers to all of the microorganisms (tiny bugs) in our bodies that are exposed to the outside surfaces. This includes the gastrointestinal organs (mouth to anus), skin, nose, ears, and genitals. These microorganisms are bacteria, protozoa, fungi, and even viruses that inhabit our bodies. It is estimated that 90 percent of cells (approximately 100 trillion cells) found in our bodies are not human, but come from 40,000 bacterial strains. Imagine, then, that we are only 10 percent human and the remainder is bugs!

Microbiome refers to the entire gene pool found in our bodies. Recall that *genes* are the instructions in cells that decide our appearances, what our personalities are like, and what health conditions we will get in our lives. Genetic material lives in all of our cells and is called our genome. There is also genetic material that comes from every bug in our guts. Some people call the gut our "second genome" or our "second brain" because of all the genetic material that comes from our bugs. Not only are the human genes outnumbered by the genetic material from our microbiota, but these gut bugs likely have a significant impact on our health as well.

The human microbiome project is a project funded by the National Institutes of Health. The project focuses on understanding the role of the microbiome in our bodies. It has given us a lot of important information on the role of the gut in how we feel and how we respond to illness. From this project, we know that the microbiota plays a critical role in building and maintaining our immune systems. Many people call the gut the "internal health monitor." It is responsible for monitoring bacteria and viruses that come into the mouth with everything we eat and preventing those infections from getting into our blood-streams and becoming systemic diseases. The gut is involved in the production of vitamins, essential amino acids, and fatty acids. It also impacts how our bodies utilize fats and sugars, which are important in understanding how we gain weight.[1] (See Consider 1.)

CONSIDER 1

☑ How does my gut bacteria contribute to my risk of illness or my risk of weight gain?

Having an intact microbiota directly impacts one's health. Similarly, having a weakened microbiota puts one's body at risk for illness. The proliferation of the wrong kind of microbiota may predispose us to autoimmune diseases, such as inflammatory bowel disease and type 1 diabetes, as well as increasing risk of obesity, infections, and depression. It also likely impacts our risk for getting allergies.[2] These microbial communities change as we age, and the type of bacteria that are present in these communities shift, based on our diets and exposures to various foods and antibiotics, which can lead to an over- or underproduction of certain microbes. Many of us believe that this second genome plays a crucial role in deciding how healthy, or how sick, we will be.

How Is the Microbiome Created?

When we are born, we go through our mothers' vaginal canals (the birth canal) and are exposed to our mothers' microbiomes. We know that when a baby is born by vaginal delivery, the bugs from the mom's vagina populate the baby's gut. We also know that if a baby is born via cesarean section, the bugs from the mom's skin populate the baby's gut. We know that the composition of the gut bugs change based on if the baby is breastfed or formula fed, whether the baby received rice cereal or was given antibiotics for an infection.[3,4] Babies then crawl on the floor and suck on their toys. They are exposed to other people, our pets, and our plants, all of which are covered in bacteria and nourish their gut. They go outside and are exposed to dirt with all of its valuable microbes. They eat the grass and lick things that our pets have licked, and they obtain more bugs. Exposure to small numbers of pathogens will strengthen our immune system. Our gut bugs also change in composition and proportion, though, depending on whether we develop an illness, on whether we take antibiotics, and on what we eat. We are just on the brink of understanding what all these changes mean and which changes are good and which ones are bad. (See Consider 2.)

CONSIDER 2

 Consider how your bacteria change depending on how you are delivered and what you are exposed to when you are young.

The Ps and Fs: Prevotella and Firmicutes

There are millions of bugs in our gut, and we don't know much about most of them. However, there do appear to be several principal types of gut bugs that change with diet in some studies. Prevotella and Firmicutes are two classes of gut bugs that change in number based on what we eat. We know that when we eat high-fat foods, we have more Firmicutes than Prevotella. When we reduce fat or carbohydrates, we increase Prevotella and decrease Firmicutes. When we eat fiber, we increase Prevotella. When we go through gastric bypass surgery, we increase Prevotella.

A study was done that looked at rural Africans and African Americans.[5] The rural Africans ate a village diet that was mostly plants, high in fiber and low in animal products. The African-American diet was high in animal fat, low in plants, and low in fiber. Interestingly, the Africans had a Prevotella predominance in their guts, and the African Americans had a Firmicutes predominance in theirs. The study went further, which is the best part. Researchers found that the African Americans had more colonic inflammation and the Africans had less. Then the researchers switched the diets of the two groups, and they found that the bacterial predominance shifted. The Africans developed a Firmicutes predominance, and the African Americans

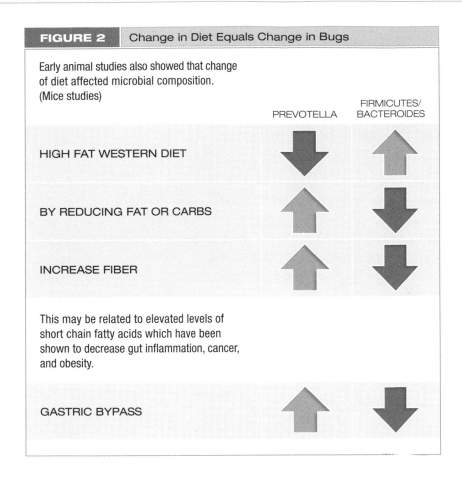

FIGURE 2   Change in Diet Equals Change in Bugs

Early animal studies also showed that change of diet affected microbial composition. (Mice studies)

	PREVOTELLA	FIRMICUTES/ BACTEROIDES
HIGH FAT WESTERN DIET	↓	↑
BY REDUCING FAT OR CARBS	↑	↓
INCREASE FIBER	↑	↓

This may be related to elevated levels of short chain fatty acids which have been shown to decrease gut inflammation, cancer, and obesity.

| GASTRIC BYPASS | ↑ | ↓ |

had a Prevotella predominance. And on top of that, colonic inflammation increased in the Africans after the diet switch and colonic inflammation decreased in the African Americans![6] How cool is that? (See figure 2.)

Short-Chain Fatty Acids

A nother important concept to note is that when bacteria break down food, they release short-chain fatty acids (SCFA). Three main SCFAs are butyrate, acetate, and propionate. We know that SCFAs are associated with decreased inflammation and are antineoplastic (anticancer causing). In the study with Africans and African Americans noted in the previous section, the Africans produced a higher number of SCFAs, which then decreased as they shifted to eating the diet lower in fiber and higher in meat! Plant-based foods were associated with higher numbers of SCFAs.[6]

Metabolites of the Gut Bugs

There are many metabolites (substances needed for metabolism or created during metabolism) that are produced by bacteria in the gut. One of those metabolites is trimethylamine N-oxide (TMAO), which is produced when foods that are high in phosphatidylcholine are ingested. The main sources of phosphatidylcholine are eggs, liver, beef, and pork. When these types of food are ingested, they are processed in the gut and the metabolites trimethylamine and TMAO are formed. In a study done at the Cleveland Clinic, researchers found that elevated levels of TMAO were associated with increased risk of major adverse cardiovascular events.[7] Much work is still needed in this area to understand the causality of this increased event rate, but, boy, it is interesting. The best part of the study to us was that the researchers also gave meat to vegetarians and vegans, and after ingestion of the food, they did not have the same increase in TMAO as the omnivores. Is this because the gut bugs in vegetarians and vegans are different from meat eaters, and, therefore, they had a different response? Much to consider here.

Another metabolite produced in the gut is lipopolysaccharide (LPS), another by-product of bacterial processing. The gut bacteria make LPS in response to a high-fat diet, which then triggers a leaky gut (more on leaky gut on pages 41–45).[8] Harmful infectious bacteria can also carry high amounts of LPS. Antibiotics that decrease bacterial overgrowth also decrease levels of LPS. Similarly, certain prebiotics (foods for gut flora) and probiotics (actual bugs that come from food or supplements) also decrease LPS. In a study of 7,000 people with diabetes, it was found that their levels of LPS were higher than in nondiabetic individuals.[9] When mice on a high-fat diet were given probiotics, their levels of insulin resistance decreased, as did their levels of LPS.[10] We know that a proportion of SCFAs similar to those in rural African children can suppress lipopolysaccharide (LPS) and other proteins that indicate inflammation (cytokine-triggered pro-inflammatory markers).[9] Importantly, high levels of LPS have also been noted in Alzheimer's disease and autism compared to healthy controls.[11,12] (See Consider 3.)

(See Consider 3.)

CONSIDER 3

 How we eat can dictate how much inflammation we produce, which is the basis for chronic illness.

The Leaky Gut

Along with gut bugs, there is more to this story that is also being revealed: leaky gut or intestinal permeability. The gut consists of the stomach, small intestine, large intestine, and rectum. It has a surface area of 3,000 square feet. It is on the surface of the gut that these microbes, or gut bugs, live. The more surface area that is present, the better our ability is to absorb and digest. The gut is also made up of an abundance of intestinal villi, which are outpouchings or protrusions in the colon that are responsible for absorption. The external layer of cells of these villi is our first line of defense, as these cells are the first to be exposed to whatever comes into the GI tract. They are the pawns on our chessboards and the infantrymen in our cavalry. (See figure 3 on the next page.)

These cells are followed by the intestinal dendritic cells, which resemble tiny trees branching out; they are often considered the first responders. These cells are the "soldiers on horses." They are more equipped to handle the entry of a pathogen. Between these cells are tight junctions, like a barricade that prevents infections from getting through. But if those junctions break and an intruder gets in, immune cells (the T and B cells) arrive, which are active immune fighters. These cells are "the snipers and our 'Navy SEALs.'" They are the best of the best, ready to attack any foreign material that invades our bodies. As Harvard professor and pediatric gastroenterologist Dr. Alessio Fasano says, "The intestinal mucosa [gut] is the battlefield on which friends and foes need to be recognized and properly managed to find the ideal balance between tolerance and immune response." Normally, when hostile bacteria and viruses come through our intestines, we have a tight junction barricade and this large cavalry to handle the enemy, and the body deals with it with hopefully few casualties.

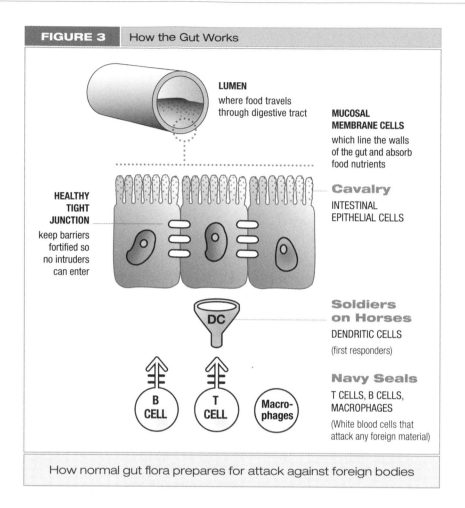

FIGURE 3 | How the Gut Works

LUMEN
where food travels
through digestive tract

MUCOSAL
MEMBRANE CELLS
which line the walls
of the gut and absorb
food nutrients

HEALTHY
TIGHT
JUNCTION
keep barriers
fortified so
no intruders
can enter

Cavalry
INTESTINAL
EPITHELIAL CELLS

DC

Soldiers
on Horses
DENDRITIC CELLS
(first responders)

B
CELL

T
CELL

Macro-
phages

Navy Seals
T CELLS, B CELLS,
MACROPHAGES
(White blood cells that
attack any foreign material)

How normal gut flora prepares for attack against foreign bodies

There are certain illnesses, however, where the tight junctions break and allow the bloodstream to be exposed to abnormal bacteria or bacterial by-products. Those abnormal by-products can then enter into the bloodstream and create an inflammatory response. A short response can be handled by the Navy SEALs without too much difficulty. But with a prolonged assault, this inflammatory response triggers formation of an abundance of inflammatory cells that can get out of hand and attack different parts of the host body.

An example of the leaky gut phenomenon is found in celiac disease, the study of which has been pioneered by Dr. Alessio Fasano. People with celiac disease have an allergy to gluten, which is present in wheat, rye, and barley. When people with gluten allergy eat gluten, their bodies respond poorly. Over time, they develop symptoms of malabsorption because their guts are unable to absorb any useful food particles—the gut is too massively inflamed. They don't just manifest gut symptoms. Inflammation rages through their bodies. They develop diarrhea, abdominal pain, skin changes, and joint pain and can have neurologic manifestations.

Note that gluten allergy is different from *gluten sensitivity*. The immune changes with gluten allergy associated with celiac disease is an autoimmune reaction. This reaction can cause damage to the lining of the intestines. Gluten sensitivity can cause many symptoms, such as headache, joint pain, and fatigue, but sensitivity doesn't necessarily damage the intestinal lining.

Dr. Fasano and others have shown that when people with gluten allergy are exposed to gluten, the tight junctions between their intestinal cells become leaky. The doors to the insides of their gut open. An environmental trigger, such as wheat in the case of celiac disease, then comes through the door and creates an immune reaction. Immune complexes form which then destroy the villi. Once destroyed, these villi cannot contribute to digestion and cannot help shunt essential nutrients into the bloodstream. Immune complexes create systemic reactions. Fasano believes that some level of leaky gut is a good thing. Most people have occasional intestinal permeability where the doors open for a short time. During that time, the immune system is exposed to foreign particles and learns to respond to them. But in celiac sufferers, the intestine is leaky for hours and the immune system becomes massively inflamed. As Fasano says, "Friend or foe: when there is a fight, there is always collateral damage, i.e., inflammation." (See figure 4 on the next page.)

Some environmental triggers can make one person have a leaky gut for hours while another person has a leaky gut for just minutes. We now know that a person must have a genetic predisposition to a certain sensitivity. We can't necessarily fix this predisposition because we get it from our parents. But it is only when the environmental trigger appears, however, that a person actually becomes sick. Then we can potentially eliminate the trigger, decrease the leaky gut, decrease inflammation, and treat the chronic disease. (See Consider 4 on page 45.)

Fasano and others believe that many autoimmune diseases are affected by food sensitivities and changes in the microbiome at an

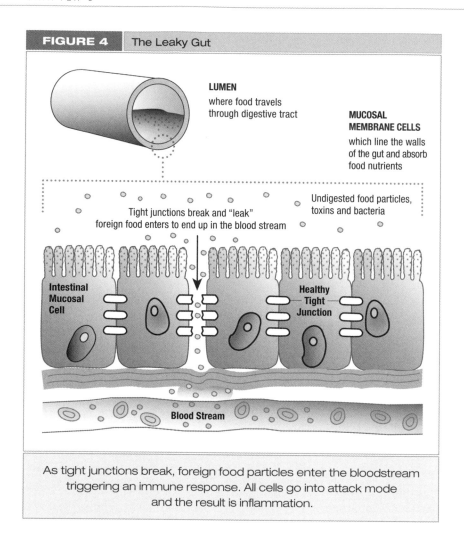

FIGURE 4 | The Leaky Gut

LUMEN
where food travels
through digestive tract

MUCOSAL MEMBRANE CELLS
which line the walls
of the gut and absorb
food nutrients

Undigested food particles,
toxins and bacteria

Tight junctions break and "leak"
foreign food enters to end up in the blood stream

Intestinal
Mucosal
Cell

Healthy
Tight
Junction

Blood Stream

As tight junctions break, foreign food particles enter the bloodstream
triggering an immune response. All cells go into attack mode
and the result is inflammation.

early age. The leaky gut has been associated with other autoimmune diseases, such as type 1 diabetes.[13] Type 1 diabetes (different from type 2 diabetes, discussed earlier) is an autoimmune disease in which someone's own immune system attacks insulin-producing beta cells. Without insulin, our bodies are unable to process sugars and convert them to storage in the form of fat. The link between how the leaky gut triggers immune reactions that attack the pancreas in some people and cause type 1 diabetes, and in others creates lupus, rheumatoid arthritis, or multiple sclerosis is not clear. Each person has different genetic predispositions and environmental triggers. Importantly, there are other environmental triggers for inflammation beside diet and gut permeability; we can't ignore the roles of stress and trauma, obesity, and smoking as important causes of total body inflammation.[8]

CONSIDER 4

 Environmental triggers can cause a leaky gut. Most of the time, a trigger is a food we eat. Food triggers are different for different people. When you eliminate a trigger, you can eliminate the inflammation.

What is unclear, however, is how much of a role the imbalance in gut bacteria has on triggering the leaky gut versus the role of genetic predisposition to some food sensitivity. In other words, will a food sensitivity alone trigger inflammation and illness in a genetically predisposed person, or do you also need dysbiosis (an unhealthy combination of gut bacteria)? We believe that you need the whole package: genetic predisposition, exposure to a sensitized food, and abnormal gut flora. Presumably, the gut flora changes based on what someone eats, and certain gut changes increase risk for a leaky gut. These gut alterations, and resulting high levels of LPS, also seem to be associated with increased intestinal permeability, and the host immune system eventually reaches a constant state of chronic inflammation.[8] In one study, mice fed a high-fat diet exhibited higher permeability to small molecules and reduced or altered junction proteins. This means that mice fed a high-fat diet could not create tight adhesions between their cells; therefore, bacterial by-products were allowed to enter their bloodstreams.[14] In chronic kidney disease patients, we see the same sort of significant bacterial overgrowth and dysbiosis, as in the mice and evidence of disruption of their intestinal barriers.[15] We believe this is what happened to Dr. A. She had a genetic predisposition to disease. She had food sensitivity to dairy and abnormal gut flora: the perfect storm.

This information is groundbreaking but still in the early stages; however, it provides clues as to the first links between changes in the microbiota and intestinal permeability. The gut likely holds the key to so many inflammatory conditions. Studies are ongoing to link high-fiber diets to increased SCFAs and determine whether that diet will reduce inflammatory conditions.

But Wait, There Is More?! The Gut-Brain Axis

There is even more to this story. While Hippocrates said back in 460 BC that all diseases begin in the gut, our understanding of its importance has been relatively recent. The gut-brain axis is a concept that was established in the 1880s and recognizes the connection between our brains and our guts, which occurs via the autonomic nervous system (the same nervous system we talked about previously). It consists of nerve branches that connect the brain to the other organsand is the control center for subconscious activity, such as breathing, swallowing, urinating, and digestion. The autonomic nervous system is divided into enteric (nervous system of the gut), sympathetic (fight or flight), and parasympathetic nervous systems (rest and recharge), which all play a role in regulating gastrointestinal function. These connections are established via the vagus nerve, which provides fibers from the brain all the way to the transverse colon. Stimulation of the vagus nerve causes not only variations in the heart rate, but also changes in gut motility. *Gut motility* is the activity of processing our food remnants into stool and removing all the important nutrients. Slow motility would suggest slow processing of food and can be witnessed as visible food contents in our stool.

As we discussed previously, when we are stressed, our sympathetic nervous systems become activated. Our senses become more acute. We see more clearly. Our hearing is more defined. We think more clearly. (See Consider 5.) Our heart rates increase so that our hearts can pump more blood to essential organs. Blood pressure increases and blood flow improves to the brain. Simultaneously, pain sensitivity is blunted, and bladder and gut motility slow down. When we are relaxed, the parasympathetic nervous system is activated. Our heart rates slow down and gut motility increases. This makes sense because if we are being chased, we need faster heart rates and elevated blood pressures. We need heightened senses and don't want to worry about having to urinate or being hungry. We can't worry about pain. When we are relaxed, our heart rates and blood pressures go down, and we become hungry. Our bowels and bladders work. We can focus on pain and deal with it. This is an important concept in gut motility, but it also becomes relevant when we talk about day-to-day stresses and ways to recharge.

CONSIDER 5

 How does acute stress affect your thinking? Consider how excess stress makes you feel. Have you ever felt like a deer caught in headlights?

While the link between the gut and brain has long been established, it is not entirely clear how the vagus nerve actually interacts with the microbiota. The link is likely related to neurotransmitters, hormones, and short-chain fatty acids that are produced by the gut. Neurotransmitters and hormones are chemical signalers or correspondents that come from the brain and travel to the gut, or vice versa. Tryptophan, for instance, is produced by the gut; it is involved in sleep function and is a main building block of protein. Serotonin, which is involved in mood, is produced in part in the gut. Most antidepressants are selective serotonin re-uptake inhibitors (SSRI), which means they prevent serotonin from breaking down. With serotonin, our moods are stabilized. Likewise, without serotonin, we suffer from depression. (See Consider 6.) Short-chain fatty acids, fatty acids produced by the gut, have been shown to improve memory and protect the brain. Only with more recent studies and ongoing research are we able to increase our understanding of the vagus nerve's true impact.

CONSIDER 6

How many people are on an SSRI, which is an antidepressant whose sole job is to increase serotonin in the body? Imagine if you healed your gut how much more serotonin you would have.

These studies on the gut-brain axis, usually done with mice, rely on a concept called "a germ-free host," an animal that theoretically has no microbiota (no gut bugs). The host mice were delivered by cesarean section, were fed sterile milk, and were raised in a sterile environment to ensure they had no microbiota. Without a microbiota, the mice experienced significantly more anxiety-related behavior, repetitive movements, and decreased memory. Biochemical and molecular changes were also noted, such as in the level of cortisol (a stress hormone) and, amazingly, the functioning of some genes. Genes that affect learning and memory were altered in germ-free hosts compared to hosts with microbiota.

Data suggests that when a normal microbiota is restored or probiotics are given to these hosts, many of the behavioral changes, such as anxiety, sociability, and other biochemical processes, can be reversed.[16] This is an amazing concept. More studies and human trials are needed.

We previously mentioned that many metabolites produced by microorganisms in the gut are also neurotransmitters in the brain. Along with serotonin and tryptophan, histamine (which is involved in immune responses) is also produced by the gut. Dopamine is a chemical messenger that causes dilation of blood vessels. Tryptophan is not only a building block of proteins, but also another neurotransmitter, serotonin, which helps us sleep. These are all important metabolites produced by the gut. Interestingly, in one study, when the guts of germ-free hosts were recolonized, the levels of serotonin and social awareness in those hosts did not change, suggesting there is an age or length of time after which gut alterations have less of an impact.

The role of the microbiota can be seen in psychiatric and neurodegenerative diseases. Autism is a neurocognitive disorder associated with decreased social skills (such as cognition) and sometimes repetitive movements. Genetic and environmental factors are believed to play a role in the development of this disease. A large number of people with autism spectrum disorder have associated gastrointestinal (GI) complaints. Studies vary, but we've learned that between 9 and 70 percent of autistic people have some GI concerns. There is recent data to suggest a link between autism spectrum disorders and the microbiota. Germ-free mice have been shown to lack social skills and have demonstrated an increase in the repetitive behaviors often seen with autism spectrum disorders.[17] Studies have shown that probiotics can decrease gut imbalance, improve these gastrointestinal complaints, and decrease immune system abnormalities. Whether probiotics can improve behavioral issues remains to be seen, and large randomized controlled trials are needed.[17]

We have now seen how our gut flora plays a very important role in how we feel. We also know that exposures from childhood are important for keeping these bugs strong and ready to attack. We have learned that in modern times the bugs in our guts have changed because of antibiotic use and perhaps highly improved sanitary conditions. (See the section on hygiene on pages 49–50.) We have shown that the foods we eat can modify our gut flora, and by-products of less nutritious foods have been linked to heart disease, Alzheimer's, and autism. We also know that a whole-grain, plant-based diet helps the composition of our microbiota to shift, so that we produce more of the SCFAs that are pivotal in maintaining a strong immune system and better overall health. Once again we see an important benefit from this diet. (See Consider 7.) All and all, the data on the microbiome is ever-expanding. We have the framework linking chronic illnesses and the microbiome, and as more of these studies are done, the treatments of chronic illness also will change.

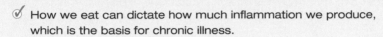

CONSIDER 7

✔ How we eat can dictate how much inflammation we produce, which is the basis for chronic illness.

We may not be able to control our genetic predispositions, but we can control our environmental triggers. We can control what we eat. Common food sensitivities believed to be triggers for leaky gut are animal products, specifically red meat, dairy products, processed foods, and gluten. All of these will be discussed later in this book. Often, treatment of many autoimmune diseases has to start through the process of elimination, discovering which environmental triggers a person is susceptible to. This concept is the foundation for diet modifications that we recommend.

Hygiene Hypothesis

anitation is very important. There is no question. Proper handwashing techniques have significantly reduced infection rates globally. Over time, however, our behaviors have changed as explained by something called the *hygiene hypothesis*. Because we are more aware of the importance of sanitation and its role in infection, we tend to clean and sterilize most everything. We know that sanitation prevents the spread of germs, and because of this knowledge, we have reduced the number of illnesses that have affected our children. But have we gone too far? Is it possible to be overly clean? What is the impact of hand sanitizers and antibacterial soaps that remove 99 percent of the bacteria on our skin? Is that a good thing? In fact, studies show that people who lived in large families in less sanitary conditions than we do today were not afflicted with the same illnesses that we are now. They had less asthma and fewer allergies.[18] Have you considered how many people you know who have a peanut allergy? In the past, this was nonexistent.

With greater access to medical care, we also take our children to doctors when they have common ailments. Often people go to their doctors' offices with colds and want antibiotics. But most of the time, these so-called colds are caused by viruses, and antibiotics are primarily ineffective against viral infections. But perhaps because of pressure from their patients, physicians will prescribe antibiotics anyway, which then disrupt their patients' gut flora. Are we doing the right thing?

Are we overtreating illnesses, and could many of them simply be monitored while our bodies' natural defenses go to work? With all of these changes in the modern era, we have also noted the onset of so many more cases of allergy, autoimmune disease, and inflammatory bowel disease.[19]

Many health professionals (and we ourselves) also assert that we should let natural things be natural. Their advice includes the following: Do not stop your kids from eating dirt, as long as it hasn't been sprayed with pesticides. Let them get dirty. Let your dog lick the kids' faces. Don't spray everything with bactericidal soap. Don't wash your hands with bactericidal soap or use alcohol-based hand sanitizers. Unless we work in a hospital or are constantly exposed to infections, the bacteria that we are exposed to are good for our microbiota. Our intestines become strong and hardy, and the intestinal barriers become strong. Nourish your bugs. Don't be afraid of them.

Probiotics

Probiotics have been defined as "live organisms that when given in adequate amounts confer health benefits."[20] Probiotics have received a great deal of attention lately. This interest started with recent studies on lactose intolerance, which is the inability of the body to break down lactose, a key component of cow's milk. As we age, the amount of lactase enzyme we produce in order to break down lactose decreases. As a result, with lactose malabsorption, people experience bloating, gas, and watery diarrhea. It has been discovered that giving those same people yogurt that contains live probiotic cultures can reduce their intolerance.[21]

Gastroenterologists and scientists have started looking at what it is about yogurt that allows people to tolerate it better than milk. In yogurt production, milk is fermented, which causes the production of lactase. Several types of bacteria are produced in yogurt cultures; two beneficial strains in particular are Lactobacillus bulgaricus and Streptococcus salivarius subsp. Thermophilus.[22] Multiple studies have shown that ingestion of variable quantities of yogurt decreases lactose malabsorption and improves tolerability. In acute diarrheal illnesses, other strains of Lactobacillus have been used for treatment.

In one important study, 287 children under three years of age with acute diarrhea were given a probiotic with oral rehydration therapy versus the rehydration therapy alone. Those who received the probiotic had shorter, less severe illnesses.[23] Also, importantly, in multiple studies, people who took probiotics while traveling were protected from traveler's diarrhea by almost 50 percent.[24] Different strains of good bacteria were used in the various studies, and a number of them were found to have benefits.

The most interesting work on probiotics extends beyond use in gut-related illnesses. In one study, pregnant women were given probiotics prior to delivery and during the period they were breastfeeding; if their babies were formula-fed, the probiotic was supplemented into the diet of the newborn. The children who had received the probiotic showed a 50 percent reduction in the amount of their eczema, and that improvement lasted for up to four years postdelivery.[25] There is also data available on decreases in dental caries (cavities) when subjects were given probiotics. Probiotics likely also play a role in improving inflammatory bowel disease.[26] Many animal studies, as well as studies done on small numbers of humans, show a role of probiotics in lessening symptoms in rheumatoid arthritis sufferers.[27,28] New studies show the potential benefits of probiotics in inflammatory overall diseases by reducing intestinal permeability and protecting against bad bugs finding a home.[29]

The action of probiotics provides us another compelling way to recognize that healing the gut heals the body. Replenishing the gut with needed healthy bacteria can decrease the overactive immune agents that develop with common infections and potentially in inflammatory diseases, such as rheumatoid arthritis and eczema and possibly inflammatory bowel disease and diabetes. Healthy gut bacteria may play a role in cancer abatement as well.

We believe that there are significant benefits to probiotics. We use them in our clinics and with our patients, depending on the case. The problem with over-the-counter probiotic supplements is that there is a lot of variability in the type and amount of bacteria that are used. Plus, there is no Food and Drug Administration safety checking of these products. We often recommend foods containing natural probiotics, such as sauerkraut, kimchi, and tempeh, to be added to the diet—especially when the gut is very sick. Think about how you can get some of these natural probiotics into your life.

Summary

1. The microbiome has a connection to the other systems in our body. It has a role in how we feel, how hungry we are, and how we respond to illness.

2. Our exposures affect the strength of our guts. We should not be afraid to get a little dirty because it nourishes our gut bugs.

3. Our diet is a trigger for many changes in the gut and puts us at a potential risk for illness.

4. Plant-based foods trigger production of more SCFAs, which are important for our immune systems and for decreasing inflammation.

5. Natural probiotics have a role in nurturing the gut.

YOUR PRESCRIPTION

1. Don't be afraid to get a little dirty.

2. Avoid hand sanitizers and use plain old soap.

3. Avoid high-fat food and meat, which trigger harmful metabolites in our bodies and have a potential role in chronic illness.

4. Avoid food triggers that create a leaky gut. Different foods will be triggers for different people, but any of them may lead to chronic illness. Be aware of what food does to your body. Eliminate one at a time and listen to your body.

5. A strong gut makes a strong body.

6. Move toward an unprocessed whole-food, plant-based diet.

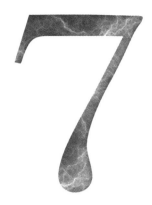

Heal Thy Gut

The role of elimination

CASE 1: Jane S is a 62-year-old female who arrived at the office with shortness of breath during exertion. She was moderately overweight with high blood pressure, very high cholesterol, and prediabetes. She wasn't active, and when she started a walking program, she was surprised that she was so short of breath. Dr. A noted her blood pressure was borderline high. Her EKG was normal, so Dr. A did a stress test, which was normal. She suggested a diet change and a cholesterol medication. The patient had heard about the memory and liver issues connected with statin medications and wanted to try changing her diet before she resorted to taking pills.

We talked about which foods she needed to eliminate. She gradually stopped eating animal fat, including dairy, over a three-month period. Her cholesterol levels came down 80 points. Her blood pressure normalized, and Dr. A started taking her off of medications. The patient lost 10 pounds. She looked fabulous and hasn't looked back.

CASE 2: Robert E is a 65-year-old man whom Dr. A has known for years. He started having rectal bleeding (bleeding out of his bottom).

He became markedly anemic (low blood count), and because of the significant anemia, he started developing exertional chest pain. Even walking to the bathroom, he would feel chest pain. He was admitted to a hospital where he required four units of blood. The doctors did an endoscopy and a colonoscopy and found diverticulosis, abnormal outpouchings in the colon which are prone to bleeding. These outpouchings cannot be fixed with medication; therefore, a high-fiber diet was recommended. During that admission, Robert also was given a stress test, which showed two areas of the heart that were receiving decreased blood flow under stress. A cardiac catheterization was recommended. Robert refused that test because he wanted to talk it over with Dr. A, his primary cardiologist, who was not involved in the proposed treatment plan. He was discharged from the hospital on multiple medications and stool softeners to improve his bowel health.

Dr. A saw no point in a catheterization because a person must be able to take blood thinners in order to be considered for a catheterization and stenting. Stents in the heart require blood thinners to ensure that the stents stay open. Then, even with stents in place, Robert would be prone to bleeding again when he was put on blood thinners because he still had untreated diverticulosis. With more bleeding, Robert would likely develop chest pain again, even with the stents in place. Dr. A believed that treating Robert would require healing the diverticulosis. She put him on a strict diet. She eliminated animal products except fish and put him on a whole-grain, plant-based diet. Three months later, Robert had had no further rectal bleeding. His blood counts had risen significantly, and he was no longer anemic. He had stopped taking his stool softeners and couldn't believe how regular his bowels were. He also no longer had any more chest pain. Six months later, Dr. A repeated a stress test, and it was normal. Flow had normalized to all parts of his heart. Amazing.

The key to good health is sometimes eliminating, rather than adding. In order to subdue or treat a chronic illness, we must minimize stresses on the body that cause inflammation. One of the most important stresses on the body is the food we take in, which can have a lasting impact on the gut. Once we fix the gut, we begin to heal. Here, we will work on how we start the healing process.

ELIMINATION #1: Remove Red Meat and Eggs
From the Diet for at Least Three Months

The first elimination that we would like people to work toward is
meat and eggs. Start with red meat. By red meat, we mean all beef,
pork, and venison in your diet, especially hot dogs and sausages. Plan
to completely rid your diet of these foods for at least three months.
This amount of time allows the gut to heal and healthy gut flora to
return, but some people will need longer to heal. After the first six
weeks of meat elimination, we recommend giving up eggs. For some,
this will be harder to give up than red meat. Try to drop eggs completely for six weeks, and then, if necessary, add them back once in a
while as a treat. The gut needs that time to heal. Eventually, we would
like you to stop eating poultry (turkey and chicken) as well. But this
can come later. One step at a time.

Why is this elimination important? Recall that red meat and
eggs cause the gut to produce TMAO (see page 40), which promotes
plaque formation in the heart. Egg yolks are also very high in cholesterol. We also know that a vegetarian diet and a high-fiber diet
are associated with decreasing TMAO.[1] Other studies link red meat
to heart disease due to the excess amount of saturated fat red meat
contains.[2] We know, too, that a high-fat diet that includes red meat
causes production of lipopolysaccharide (LPS, see page 40). Recall
that LPS is responsible for dysbiosis and a leaky gut and is found in
abundance in many sufferers of chronic illness. Red meat, then, is a
trigger for inflammation.

What else do we know about the detrimental effects of meat? The
salt in meat can be linked to high blood pressure. Nitrates, which are
used as preservatives in meat, have been associated with poor dilation
of the blood vessels (endothelial dysfunction) and insulin resistance.[3,4]
On the other hand, we know from the early work of Dean Ornish,
MD, that patients with heart disease who are put on a low-fat, plant-
based diet had less plaque in their heart arteries.[43] Dr. Ornish is a
Harvard-trained physician who pioneered much of the early work
on plant-based diet and heart disease. We also know from Caldwell
Esselstyn's recent work at the Cleveland Clinic that adhering to a
strictly plant-based diet can reduce plaque and increase blood flow to
previously restricted areas.[5] (See figure 1 on the next page.)

FIGURE 1	Negative Health Effects of Meat and Eggs

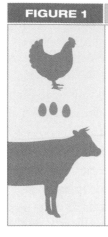

Eating red meat and eggs can cause the gut to:

- Produce TMAO—which promotes plaque formation in the heart.
- Elevate saturated fats—linked to heart disease
- Increase production of lipopolysaccharide—leading to dybiosis of the gut—causing leaky gut and inflammation
- Elevate levels of salt—linked to high blood pressure
- Increase nitrate levels—endothelial dysfunction and insulin resistance
- Elevate heterocyclic amines—increase free radicals—increase risk of cancer

Red meat is also associated with increased risk of many cancers.[2] Nitrate-derived metabolites, polycyclic aromatic hydrocarbons, and heterocyclic amines (HCAs) are all possible carcinogens (cancer causing) and are found in red meat.[6] Meat that is grilled is cooked at high temperatures. When that meat darkens on the grill and is well done, HCAs are produced and appear to cause cancer. Even the excess iron in red meat may trigger some of these potential carcinogens.[7] Red meat is also thought to be a cause of oxidative stress, which, as you may recall, is a stressor on the system that triggers the formation of free radicals that are believed to be the starting point for cancer.[2]

The data is compelling regarding this elimination. Red meat and eggs should be eliminated. We know this seems drastic. However, the impact of illness cannot be underestimated. These changes can happen, and if you want to be healthy, you must make them. Our recommendation is to start slowly, but deliberately.

What about fish and poultry? Eventually, we think we should eliminate at least all of the chicken we eat. People are focused on chicken as a healthier option than red meat, and while it may be a slightly healthier option, it is not all that healthful. Intake of chicken has grown significantly since the 1980s, and the consumption of red meat has gone down by 30 percent, but chronic illnesses persist and continue to increase. Chicken is still too inflammatory for our bodies; it's also high in cholesterol and produces TMAO. We know this is tough love, but as heart-health expert Dr. Caldwell Esselstyn says, "Moderation kills." After red meat and eggs, we recommend eliminating all chicken from our diets. Fish is the only food for which we have substantial evidence of lowering the risk of sudden death and coronary heart disease, probably due to its abundance of omega-3 fatty acids (more on fatty acids on pages 93–96).[8,9] Data suggests that eating two or more servings of fatty fish per week (mackerel, salmon, tuna) is associated with a decreased risk of heart disease. While we are not fish eaters, there is some evidence to support its benefit, so if you want to keep any meat, keep the fish.

It is interesting to note that the Tarahumara Indians of Mexico are known as wellness warriors, because they are extremely active mountain runners and have virtually no coronary artery disease (heart disease clogs). Their diet is at least 90 percent beans and maize. Ninety-four percent of their protein comes from vegetable sources; only 6 percent is from animal sources. Of their fat intake, 33 percent is from vegetables and 67 percent comes from animals.[10] Most of their sources of vegetables are corn and beans. Their cholesterol is derived from two eggs per week and rare servings of meat. The main source of calcium is corn tortillas made on limestone slabs, so the tortillas absorb some of the calcium from the limestone.[10]

Are we saying there is no room for an occasional meat dish? That's a difficult question. We know that eating meat is not good for our bodies. After three months of healing the microbiome, can our bodies tolerate a little meat? Perhaps—it's hard to say for sure. Dr. A knows that with her chronic illness, she doesn't have room for "maybe." She feels that she has to be as close to perfect as possible because she doesn't want to get sick again. Can others who don't have a chronic illness still have some flexibility? Consider that heart disease is insidious. One-third of people with heart disease who die suddenly had no previous symptoms. We have to consider someone's risk factors and determine what level of flexibility exists. (See Consider 1.)

CONSIDER 1

✓ Plan for three months of no meat or eggs, which allows time for the gut to heal. After that, is there room for an occasional meat or egg dish? Maybe, we don't know. Everyone's body will respond differently.

At the same time, we would also say that everyone is doing their best. Eating less is always better than eating more. Do the best you can. Set goals and focus. You can do this. Consider the alternative: feeling bad, miserable even, and having a chronic illness. Isn't a healthy, meat-free diet worth a try?

This is difficult for many people; they tell us they have eaten meat and potatoes their whole lives and can't imagine never eating them again. We always remind them that elimination is hard, but taking medications is hard too. What would you do if it meant you could stop taking medicine? What would you give up to live a longer, healthier life?

ELIMINATION #2: Eliminate Dairy—All of It.

Dairy refers to foods that come from cows. So removing dairy means removing cow's milk, cheese, and butter. Once milk is obtained from cows on farms, it is pasteurized. Pasteurization is the process of heating something to high temperatures, then cooling it quickly; the goal is to kill microorganisms that develop and spoil milk in order to give the product a longer shelf life.

Pasteurization works. It enables us to transfer milk from farms to grocery stores, so it will keep for 10 days after opening. Before pasteurization, dairy would be full of harmful bacteria by the time it got to the table, and children were getting sick from drinking it. Pasteurization is done to avoid that bacteria from forming, given the distance milk must travel and the time that passes before we actually drink it.

With pasteurization, however, we not only remove bacteria, but we also kill enzymes that we need to break down milk in our bodies.[11] When these enzymes are destroyed, our bodies are not as equipped to process milk. Many of us are sensitive to milk and have a milk allergy or milk sensitivity because we lack the enzyme lactase. But we believe these dairy products also trigger a leaky gut.[12] As dairy products enter the gut, the tight junctions break and the breakdown products of milk enter the bloodstream. Our immune systems are activated, and our bodies develop immune complexes that start attacking parts of the body. (See figure 2.)

We know that chronic inflammation increases risk for heart disease and cancer. In some studies, when dairy was replaced with a

FIGURE 2	Negative Health Effects of Milk
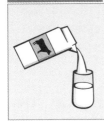	Consequences of milk sensitivity: ▪ Leaky Gut—leads to inflammation ▪ Galactose ingestion—which decreases cognitive function, decreases immune function, increases oxidative stress ▪ Suggestion of potential increased fracture risk

plant-based protein source, there was a reduction in cardiovascular disease![13] Inflammation is also a trigger for bone breakdown. Suggesting, then, that we drink more milk to decrease our fracture risk is a "conceivable contradiction."[14] There are many studies that suggest a link between increased dairy and cardiovascular risk.[15,16] In a follow-up to these initial mouse studies, an extensive review was conducted to evaluate human milk intake. One of the studies in that review evaluated people who drank more than three glasses of milk per day versus those who drank fewer than one glass per day. The research found higher fracture and death rates in women who drank more milk. There was also a higher rate of death in men who drank more milk, though the fracture rate was not significantly different. Markers of inflammation and oxidative stress were also higher in those who drank more milk.[14]

In the 12-year Nurses' Health Study, nurses who drank more than two glasses of milk per day had no fewer fractures than those nurses consuming less than one glass of milk per week.[17] Interestingly, in that same study, those who consumed greater amounts of calcium from dairy foods had a higher fracture risk. That increased risk was not seen with calcium from nondairy sources.[17]

This is really important. In other corroborating research, a meta-analysis of multiple larger trials showed there was no decrease in hip fractures with calcium supplementation.[18] This means that taking calcium supplements did not decrease the rate of fractures. There may even have been a slightly higher fracture risk in people taking calcium supplements who didn't get adequate vitamin D.

Let's consider the occurrence of fractures around the world. In countries such as India, Japan, and Peru, calcium intake is less than one-third of the US daily recommended allowance (300 milligrams per day), and the risk of fractures in those countries is extremely low. The countries with the highest fracture risks are actually those where people drank an abundance of milk, namely Norway, Sweden, Iceland, Denmark, and the US. These studies suggest that maybe drinking milk is not all it's cracked up to be! (See Consider 2.)

CONSIDER 2

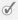 People who live in countries where less milk is consumed have fewer fractures.

We also note that people with high-sodium and high-protein diets absorb less calcium and excrete more calcium in their urine.[19] In the Nurses' Health Study, those nurses who took in more than 95 grams of protein per day were 20 percent more likely to fracture a bone than those who ingested less than 68 grams per day.[20] It is suspected that people with a diet lower in protein and sodium likely need less calcium in their diets. Protein from meat and eggs contains high concentrations of sulfate amino acids, which can cause calcium losses in the urine. Vegetarian diets are typically lower in protein than nonvegetarian diets. Notably, however, both groups in the Nurses' Health Study exceeded the recommended daily allowance for protein (RDA). This may explain why people in countries where less red meat and fat are typically eaten require less calcium.

We believe that building bones requires many components. We know that calcium is very important to bone development, but we don't know how much calcium we need or the proper means for getting calcium into our systems. Besides a diet rich in calcium, we know it is essential to have an abundance of vitamins D and K. In the Nurses' Health Study, researchers actually found an increase in fracture risk in women who consumed dairy sources for calcium versus those who consumed nondairy sources of calcium. (See figure 3.)

Calcium comes from many nondairy sources, including broccoli, kale, collard greens, turnip greens (6 ounces contain 220 milligrams calcium), bok choy, almonds (3 ounces have 210 milligrams), sunflower seeds, tahini, dried beans, and blackstrap molasses. Flaxseeds and sesame seeds are two more great sources of calcium.[21] Calcium in low-

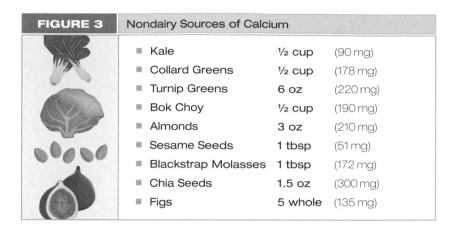

FIGURE 3	Nondairy Sources of Calcium		
	Kale	½ cup	(90 mg)
	Collard Greens	½ cup	(178 mg)
	Turnip Greens	6 oz	(220 mg)
	Bok Choy	½ cup	(190 mg)
	Almonds	3 oz	(210 mg)
	Sesame Seeds	1 tbsp	(51 mg)
	Blackstrap Molasses	1 tbsp	(172 mg)
	Chia Seeds	1.5 oz	(300 mg)
	Figs	5 whole	(135 mg)

oxalate vegetables, such as kale, is readily absorbed, so they are viable options for calcium intake in a plant-based diet.[22] (See Consider 3.)

CONSIDER 3

☑ Spinach is rich in calcium, but it's mostly in the form of calcium oxalate, which may actually cause you to lose calcium in your urine and too much may predispose you to kidney stones. Eat spinach for iron and vitamins but not necessarily for calcium. Eat low oxalate vegetables for calcium.

Vitamin D

Vitamin D is also very important for bone health. It helps us to absorb calcium and not lose it when we urinate. Vitamin D is produced by the skin when we are exposed to sunlight. However, winter sun is not strong enough in regions above 40 degrees latitude (north of Philadelphia and San Francisco) to aid in converting vitamin D to its active form. Sunscreens, while effective for preventing sun damage, inhibit the production of vitamin D. Therefore, many of us are vitamin D deficient, regardless of whether we drink milk or not. Cow's milk does *not* have vitamin D in it, so we fortify it with vitamin D. Similarly, almond milk also is fortified with vitamin D. We have data to suggest that vitamin D (700 to 800 IU) is a daily dose that lowers the risk of hip fracture in adults.[23] This is not the same for children, and childrens' dosing should be discussed with a pediatrician.

Vitamin K

V itamin K is another important vitamin for bone health. Data shows that taking in less than 110 micrograms of vitamin K daily can increase your fracture risk. In the Nurses' Health Study, those who ate a serving of greens every day experienced only half the fractures of those who ate just one serving per week.[24] The Framingham Heart Study corroborated this idea.[25] Broccoli, kale, brussels sprouts, and collard greens are good sources of vitamin K.

Other substances in our diets may also raise our risk of osteoporosis. Excess coffee and caffeine may increase the kidneys' ability to remove calcium from the bloodstream. In the Framingham Osteoporosis Study, older women who drank caffeinated soda had a higher incidence of fractures than those who did not.[26]

Bottom Line: We have no data to suggest that dairy is needed to lower our risk of osteoporosis. We do need calcium, but we don't need much. We also need vitamins D and K to help calcium build bone density. The goal should be to eat calcium-rich, nondairy products. Guidelines recommend people below the age of 50 get 1,000 milligrams of calcium daily and postmenopausal women 1,200 milligrams daily. However, there is no scientific data to confirm that drinking cow's milk is better than the alternatives. We need to focus on a diet with lots of calcium-rich greens (also rich in vitamin K) and an adequate dose of vitamin D daily.

What About Milk and Cancer?

S tudies suggest a correlation between milk intake and bladder and prostate cancer, as well as a potential link to colon cancer.[27] There are connections between galactose and ovarian cancer. This association was found in women who drank more than three glasses of milk per day.[28] In a Harvard study of male professionals, men who drank more than two glasses of milk per day had an increased risk of prostate cancer compared to those who did not drink milk.[29] In another study, men who consumed more than 2,000 milligrams of calcium suffered almost double the rate of fatal prostate cancer than those who did not. There has been much speculation about the increased risks of reproductive cancers from drinking milk produced from cows that were injected with different hormones to produce excess milk.[30] Recent studies have also linked milk to an increase in acne, which may be related to the hormones in milk.[31]

T. Colin Campbell, author of *The China Study*, also feels that over-consumption of animal-based proteins can be detrimental to health. He specifically conducted rat and mice studies that showed a 20 per-cent casein (milk protein) diet promoted liver cancer in the animals, and when the animals were fed a reduced-casein diet of 5 percent, their tumor growth was reduced. Even when the diet was switched from high to low casein, the results were the same—reduced casein resulted in less tumor growth. Animals that consumed a diet containing 20 percent casein were all dead at 100 weeks.[32] Even though these studies are based on rats and mice, they point to a possible concern about consuming too much casein.

What About Milk and Autoimmune Disease?

Milk has been linked to inflammation and oxidative stress.[33] How milk triggers inflammation is not entirely clear. However, it is likely through a leaky gut (see pages 41–45). In some people, milk is like gluten, triggering breakdown of the tight junctions and allowing food products to enter the bloodstream. These food products prompt an attack from our gut defense system, bringing on a full inflammatory response: a body on fire. Dr. A believes strongly that dairy triggered her leaky gut and caused the autoimmune reaction of her disease. Eliminating milk products healed her.

What About Yogurt and Sour Milk?

It is important to note that in studies, the same level of inflamma-tion was not noted when people drank sour milk or ate yogurt. In fact, a negative relationship was found; i.e., sour milk and yogurt did not increase inflammation and may actually decrease inflammation.[33] These findings may be related to the fact that there is little to no lactose and galactose in these fermented products, and they may also have pro-biotic antioxidant and anti-inflammatory benefits.[34] More study is required on yogurt and fermented milk products. Likely, they do not have the same effect on the body as other milk products. If you have to choose milk products, these are the ones to choose.

Milk in Our Daily Life

There is a great deal of data that suggests that people live shorter lives when they drink milk, and most notably, they do *not* have fewer fractures. The popular conception that milk helps build strong bones needs to be reconsidered and modified. Dr. A's children have been told that they're eating a bad diet because it does not have milk in it. If they buy a school lunch, they are required to take milk. When we look at the healthy school meal, it always includes milk. Are we teaching our kids the right thing?

The American diet has butter and cheese in almost everything. If you get a side of black beans at a Mexican restaurant, there is always a sprinkle of cheddar cheese on it. If you get a salad, you usually get a sprinkle of mozzarella or Parmesan. Pasta sauces and soups have cream in them. This elimination is hard, no question, and takes education and effort. However, once you feel better, your sacrifice will be worth it.

So, start by removing the milk from the house. Buy almond or soy milk instead; there are many brands on the market these days, including unsweetened and unflavored options. Try to drink the ones in the refrigerated section because they contain fewer additives. You can even buy chocolate almond milk, which is delicious.

Instead of butter, which is made with cow's milk, switch to a plant-based margarine with plant sterols and no partially hydrogenated oils. Or better yet, avoid all butters all together! You won't notice the difference when you switch to plant-based margarines, and eventually you won't miss it at all if you stop using it all together. You also can find coconut, soy, and almond milk yogurts.

Get rid of your cheese and replace it with plant-based cheese alternatives as a transition. These options don't taste quite the same as dairy cheese, but many of them melt, shred, and spread just like dairy cheese. Eventually, you can move to no cheese at all. Personally, Dr. A would rather not eat cheese now at all. It seems strange to her that she doesn't miss it when she was so addicted to dairy for so long. You will get there too! (See figure 4 and Consider 4.)

Are We Getting Enough Protein?

eople often become highly concerned about getting sufficient protein and calcium in a diet that includes no dairy, eggs, or

FIGURE 4	Alternatives to Cow's Milk
	▪ soy milk and yogurt ▪ cashew cream ▪ almond milk and yogurt ▪ nut cheese ▪ coconut milk and yogurt

meat. This is what we are asked the most: how will I get my protein on such a diet? For those just starting their transitions and still eating chicken and fish, protein sources are evident. To those of you who have taken it to the next level and completely eliminated all animal products, we promise that you will get enough protein! People don't become protein deficient anymore unless they are truly starving. Some of the best athletes in the world eat completely plant-based diets. Dr. A did her first triathlon after going completely plant-based. You will have plenty of energy. In fact, you probably will have more energy than before on a diet of plant-based foods and (as we teach you to eat things that are minimally processed) foods with no added sugar.

CONSIDER 4

☑ Next time you are ordering pizza at a restaurant or even takeout, ask them to hold the cheese. Try it; you might be surprised, and every place we have ever eaten will make this for you.

ELIMINATION #3: Processed Foods

Processed foods are those that have been altered from their natural state. This refers to any food that has been canned, frozen, dehydrated, pasteurized, or changed by other means.

Is processing a bad thing? Often, we process foods to make them last longer by canning, freezing, or dehydrating them. That is not necessarily a bad thing. It allows for many conveniences. We pasteurize food to kill harmful bacteria, so it can last longer on our shelves. However, pasteurization often destroys heat-sensitive nutrients, as well. Many processed foods include an abundance of saturated fats, oils, and salt. Oily, fried, and fatty products last longer. The problem is that excess fats and oils put us at risk for cardiovascular disease, and excess sodium increases risk of high blood pressure.

We also process foods by adding preservatives to make them last longer. Sometimes sodium is used to preserve foods, such as with deli meats, and at other times artificial preservatives are added. Preservatives and artificial flavors are often highly inflammatory, and initiate a spiral toward chronic illness. Many foods also contain high-fructose corn syrup, an artificial sweetener. Corn syrup was introduced into the food market decades ago because sugar was so expensive. There was an abundance of corn, and corn syrup was easy and inexpensive to make. Now, corn syrup is in a huge percentage of products in the United States—even in ketchup! The problem with high-fructose corn syrup is that it is a processed, unnatural sweetener; therefore, we believe it could be inflammatory. It also blocks our natural desire to stop eating and prevents us from feeling full.

Consider how much of our food comes in a bag or lasts on the shelf for weeks on end. Food shouldn't last that long. It should go bad, and food without excess processing and preservatives will. There is no question that we need to preserve foods to get through harsh winters and travel. Canning and dehydrating are great options for this.

Another form of processing is the manufacture of refined foods. Often food we buy has gone from being whole-grain to a thin remnant of its former self. Consider oatmeal. Whole-grain oats are large and thick, at least one to two millimeters thick. When you buy instant oatmeal, the oats are only a tenth that thick. They have been shaved down so they can be cooked in 30 seconds in the microwave and are easier to eat, but all of the benefits of its fiber content are gone. Our breads are similar. Our wheat has been thinned and broken down and then made into bread. This makes the bread easier to eat, but we have lost all the benefits of the product. This is what has given bread a bad name. Refined products have minimal fiber and little nutritional value. We want our food to have bulk. That bulk is good for digestion and good for increasing the density of food in our stomachs; it's what makes us feel full.

When we first started eliminating processed foods, we began by saying we wouldn't eat food that was sold in a bag. That is difficult these days, when half the food in the grocery store is bagged. We started buying our bread in the bakery section of the supermarket, where the breads often don't have artificial preservatives in them. We now go grocery shopping a few times a week. We buy fresh food and eat it for a few days until we finish it. Then we go back for more. People often say they are too busy to go to the grocery store more than once per week, but we find that life is simpler now. We buy fresh food, cook it, and enjoy it. The flavors that come from fresh foods are one of a kind.

A Note on Canned Foods

Canned foods are preserved but very practical, especially in the winter. While we encourage eating fresh foods, that is not always possible. Look for canned foods that have only salt in them as a preservative, such as beans and vegetables. Wash the beans thoroughly, which removes about one-third of the sodium.

Another great option for beans and legumes is dried beans. There are no preservatives in these. You do have to plan ahead before using them, though, because dried beans and legumes often require soaking for several hours or overnight before cooking. Slow cookers and pressure cookers are more efficient than simmering beans on a stove top and will save considerable time. (See Consider 5.)

CONSIDER 5

✓ Canned foods are not the enemy. Ideally, we don't eat canned vegetables but eat them fresh. Canned beans are very useful in a busy household, however. Canned foods do have salt in them as a preservative, which is the negative. Salt restriction is most important for people with heart failure, and some restriction is necessary if they have high blood pressure. Most people, though, can tolerate canned beans without difficulty. Rinse them thoroughly, and that will remove about a third of the salt.

ELIMINATION #4: Sugars—Our Newest Addiction

Processed sweeteners are the most common food additives worldwide. In 2009, Americans consumed an average of more than 130 pounds of processed sweeteners a year![35] That translates to an average of one-third of a pound (about 5.7 ounces, 160 grams, or 36 teaspoons) of processed sweeteners each day, per person. This consumption is almost seven times the American Heart Association guidelines of

24 grams of processed sugar per day for women (approximately 6 tea-spoons, which is a little less than 1 ounce) and more than four times the 36 grams per day recommended for men (about 9 teaspoons).[36] For a very simple example, one 12-ounce soda contains an average of about 40 grams of added sugars, well in excess of the recommended daily sugar intake.

Artificial sweeteners exist because they are supposedly low-calorie alternatives to sugar. People think that when they drink their coffee with artificial sweeteners, they won't gain weight. But is that true? In one population-based study, 474 people were followed for almost 10 years. Those participants who drank diet soda had a 70 percent higher increase in waist circumference than consumers who didn't. Those who drank two or more diet sodas per day reported a shocking 500 percent increase in waist circumference over consumers who drank something other than diet soda![37]

Another study was done on rats that were fed the artificial sweetener aspartame. They subsequently showed an increase in blood glucose without a decrease in insulin-producing cells, suggesting insulin resistance. This study suggested that drinking diet soda could be a risk for developing diabetes.[38]

FIGURE 5	Alternatives to Artificial Sweeteners
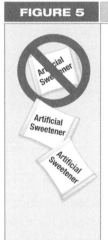	Don't use artificial sweeteners. They don't make you lose weight and likely make you gain weight. They are also inflammatory. First try your coffee/tea without any sugar at all! You will get used to it over time. Sugar is a drug and with time and slow weaning, you won't miss it. Before you get to the "no added sugar" option, try these options while you wean: ▪ Dates—great in cooking, super sweet ▪ Blueberries—great in cooking, super sweet ▪ Applesauce ▪ Cane sugar (regular sugar) ▪ Honey The Bottom Line: we would rather you eat sugar than an artificial sweetener.

A more recent study in 2013 showed that diet drinks contribute to obesity.[39] A recent article in *Nature* linked artificial sweeteners with dysbiosis (disruption of the microbiome) and increased insulin resistance (prediabetes).[40] These studies show that artificial sweeteners are not better and are likely worse. We do not believe in diet drinks. They worsen the obesity problem and should be completely avoided. We are only fooling ourselves if we drink them. (See figure 5.)

Most processed foods are bad for us. Cookies and cakes sit on store shelves for weeks, full of preservatives so they stay moist. Artificial sweeteners are added to our foods so they can be labeled as "zero calorie." Artificial sweeteners are chemicals, and they make us sick. Learn to read labels and don't eat processed foods.

Consider that if you want to eat cookies, make them yourself. Add fresh sugar, or change to dates, applesauce, and bananas for sweetening foods. Buy fresh ingredients, and you won't go wrong. Make pumpkin bread and cornbread using a mix, but just change the egg to applesauce with baking powder (one egg equals four

FIGURE 6	Alternatives in Baking

Egg Alternatives

1. Tofu can be used as a "egg" scramble—
   ¼ cup of puréed tofu = 1 egg

2. Applesauce, used in baking—
   ¼ cup applesauce with 1 teaspoon of baking powder = 1 egg

3. Potato starch—2 tbsp potato starch = 1 egg

4. Prunes—¼ cup pureed prunes = 1 egg

5. Flax seeds need to soak and becomes good binder—
   1 tbsp ground flax with 3 tbsp water, leave to soak for 5 minutes

6. Banana—½ banana = 1 egg

Dairy Alternatives

1. Consider almond or soy milk

2. Soy cheese alternatives

3. Blended cashews make a nice cream salad dressing or creamy cheese with nutritional yeast

4. Soy or coconut milk yogurts

ounces of applesauce and one teaspoon of baking powder) and cow's milk to coconut milk. You will need less oil when you use applesauce. If you want pizza, make the dough yourself and use red sauce with an abundance of vegetables. Skip the cheese! Yum. (See figure 6 on the previous page.)

What Other Harmful Foods Do We Eat?

Too many of us have absolutely no idea what is in our food. Often we see words on the ingredient lists that we've never heard of, but we just accept that they are safe to eat. Most of what we eat comes in a package, and we have no contact with the source of our food.

Reading the ingredient list can be intimidating, so most people don't even bother looking at it. We hope that after reading the information presented here, you will become a real nutrition label detective, reading and evaluating all of the ingredients in any packaged food before you purchase it.

Part of the problem is that we have lost that connection with our food. Many city dwellers in America today haven't seen how fresh food is grown. We often don't know how foods grow in their native climates. Most of us definitely do not grow our own. Home-cooked meals made with fresh ingredients are rarities in many households. We rely on packaged foods, restaurant meals, and fast food.

We also expect the government and food industry to protect us from potentially harmful ingredients. But are they really protecting us? In eating mostly processed foods, we are regularly exposed to food products that are not natural to the human body, including

- genetically modified organisms (GMOs);
- artificial colorings and flavorings;
- high-fructose corn syrup and artificial sweeteners;
- processed fats, including hydrogenated oils and even trans fats;
- naturally occurring saturated fats from animals often eating GMO feed;
- fertilizers and pesticides;
- overprocessed refined grains;

■ and animal products that can contain drugs, including antibiotics and growth hormones.

Genetically Modified Organisms (GMOs)

G MOs are plants or animals that have been genetically altered by inserting genes from foreign bacteria, viruses, insects, and other sources into the DNA of the host plant or animal. Originally introduced into our food supply in the 1990s, GMOs in plants typically are genetic modifications that allow the plant to either withstand heavy applications of pesticides or actually produce pesticides in the plant itself. The inserted genes are from living organisms that have different DNA from the original food or animal. There has been no requirement by the government for any testing to prove the safety of genetically modified foods for human consumption. We have only the manufacturer's claim that these foods are safe for human consumption. In the United States, we currently have no labeling laws requiring food manufacturers to label GMO foods, so you do not even know when you are consuming a genetically altered product. The majority of corn and soy produced in America is genetically modified.

The main upside to GMO crops is that we have created a more durable product that can potentially increase the yield of food. This is an important benefit for a rapidly growing world population. However, there is significant concern that genetically altering food affects how our bodies deal with it, creating inflammation and triggering chronic illness. A variety of animal studies implicate GMOs as potential health hazards, but very few human studies have been completed. One human study, completed in Canada in 2011, discovered some of the pesticides associated with GMO foods were found in the blood of both pregnant and nonpregnant women in Canada.[41] This is concerning, but the true impact on the body is not known.

The American Academy of Environmental Medicine suggested to its members in 2008 that they educate their patients about the potential health dangers of GMOs.[42] Overall, we recommend trying to avoid genetically modified foods. This can be done by choosing organic foods. The most common genetically modified foods are corn, soybeans, and canola and cottonseed oils. Tomatoes and potatoes are also often genetically modified, as well as papaya.

COMMIT TO ELIMINATION

Know you can do this. Elimination will cleanse your body and heal your microbiome.

- Start with eliminating red meat for six weeks.
- After six weeks, eliminate eggs, especially egg yolk, the source of cholesterol in eggs.
- After six more weeks, start replacing foods from cow's milk with plant-based alternatives.
- By three months, move toward eliminating chicken.
- Eliminate highly processed foods. Think natural.
- Cut out added sugars and fake sugars.
- Eat fresh.
- Go to the grocery store a few times per week.
- Go to a bakery for your bread.
- If you want to eat cookies, bake them yourself.

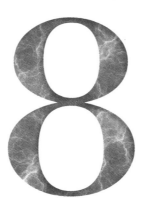

Superfoods

GREENS, BEANS, CARBS, OH MY!

Adding back

When Dr. A was younger, she constantly battled her weight. She always felt overweight and worried. She ate diet bars and drank Diet Coke. She starved herself at times and weighed herself at least once a day, but usually would feel disappointed. We know the feeling when nothing fits or the feeling of not wanting to take your shirt off at the swimming pool to show off your body. After Dr. A had her three children and got so sick, she learned how to eat. Dr. A and Dr. R don't eat any weight-reducing foods. They just eat healthily and feel great.

In the previous chapter, we spent a lot of time talking about which foods to take out of the diet—toxins—to allow for gut healing. As with everything, we have to balance that by adding back resources for the body—foods that replenish and restore. This chapter will focus on replenishment of resources, which is as important as what we eliminate.

ADD BACK #1: Fruits and Vegetables

The importance of fruits and vegetables has been purported for centuries. Fruits contain vitamins A and C, as well as potassium. Vegetables give us an abundance of fiber, vitamins A and C, iron, magnesium, calcium, and potassium. They even have protein. Fruits and vegetables are rich in phytonutrients (plant nutrients) and plant sterols (discussed on page 102). These phytonutrients have been shown in many trials to be beneficial. In times of acute stress, phytonutrients activate stress signals, which are important in cell defense.[1] Then phytonutrients arm us with defenses against damage and illness. Phytonutrients are also antioxidants. You may recall that oxidation occurs with prolonged distress and triggers free radicals that are cancer promoting and increase inflammation. The antioxidant effect of phytonutrients, then, is to decrease inflammation.

Phytonutrients can be broken down into important components, such as carotenoids, flavonoids, resveratrol, and phytoestrogens. The more brightly colored the fruits and vegetables, the more abundant they are in these components. Different vegetables have different phytonutrients in them, which is why people often say to "eat the rainbow." (See figure 1.) Red vegetables, such as tomatoes, are known for containing lycopene, which is believed to lower men's risk of prostate cancer.[2] Recent data suggests it may also reduce our risk of strokes.[3] Orange fruits and vegetables, such as oranges and pumpkins, have beta carotene, among other components. Beta-carotene may bring added benefits because it is converted to vitamin A. Beta-carotenoids, such as lutein and zeaxanthin, are found in most vegetables and in abundance in our green leafy vegetables.

These vitamin A precursors (substances that can be converted into vitamin A) are also found in abundance in our eyes and appear to protect against eye diseases.[4] Blue-colored fruits, such as grapes, red wine, and blueberries, are rich in flavonoids, such as resveratrol, which is a potent antioxidant and appears to have a role in dilating (opening up) blood vessels and may help with decreasing risk of heart disease.[5,6,7] It also has a potential antiaging effect, as shown in mice studies. Human studies, however, are inconclusive.[7] Since not all fruits and vegetables possess all the phytonutrients, it is important to eat a variety of colors to ensure you are getting all of the health benefits.

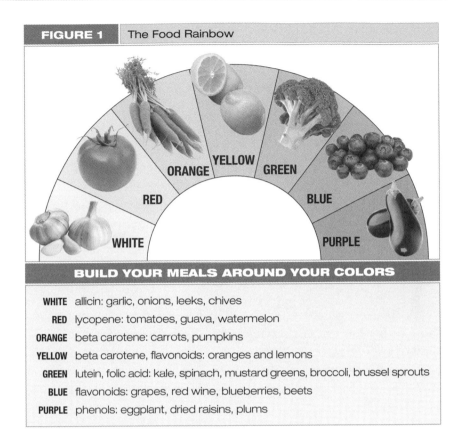

FIGURE 1   The Food Rainbow

YELLOW

ORANGE   GREEN

RED   BLUE

WHITE   PURPLE

BUILD YOUR MEALS AROUND YOUR COLORS

WHITE	allicin: garlic, onions, leeks, chives
RED	lycopene: tomatoes, guava, watermelon
ORANGE	beta carotene: carrots, pumpkins
YELLOW	beta carotene, flavonoids: oranges and lemons
GREEN	lutein, folic acid: kale, spinach, mustard greens, broccoli, brussel sprouts
BLUE	flavonoids: grapes, red wine, blueberries, beets
PURPLE	phenols: eggplant, dried raisins, plums

How Much Is Enough?

ver the centuries, the benefits of fruits and vegetables have long been purported. However, it has been unclear how many servings are really enough. In 1990, the World Health Organization decided to quantify a recommended amount. At that time, they recommended a minimum intake of 400 grams of fruits and vegetables per day to decrease the risk of cardiovascular disease and cancer.[8] Shortly after, the idea of five servings of fruits and vegetables per day was adopted by the United Kingdom and subsequently by France and Germany. The United States then adopted a more-is-better stance, and it became widely accepted that fruits and vegetables should be encouraged.

But there has been much debate about how effective fruits and vegetables are in combating chronic illness. Their role in reducing cardiovascular illness has been shown in multiple meta-analyses (large studies that assemble an overview of many smaller studies) and is quite compelling, but whether they lower cancer risk has been less clear.[9] In 2013, a study was published that showed when we eat more fruits and vegetables, we live longer.[10] This relationship was most notable in relation to reduction in cardiovascular deaths (heart disease). In this same study, the relationship was more compelling for raw vegetables than cooked. (See Consider 1.)

CONSIDER 1

☑ When we eat more fruits and vegetables, we live longer! Don't think so much about which fruit or vegetable is better; all are good. Eat them often and in quantity.

A 2014 British analysis showed a significant survival benefit for those eating one to three servings of fruits and vegetables versus less than one serving per day.[11] However, the survival benefit was highest in those who ate more than seven servings per day. Further, this study showed that the benefits were most notable with higher intake of different varieties of vegetables, salads, fresh fruit, and dried fruit. Canned and frozen fruit consumption also conferred a survival benefit. In this study, however, canned and frozen fruits were lumped together, and the benefit of each individually could not be assessed. Please note, however, that canned and dried fruits often have a significantly higher sugar content than frozen fruits.

While some studies suggest vegetables are more important to overall survival, other studies have shown that fruits are better.[12] We feel there is enough data to suggest that they are both good. People often ask which fruits and vegetables are the most beneficial. We tell them that it doesn't matter; they are all good. However, the ratio likely should be closer to two vegetables per one fruit.

Fruits have more simple sugars, such as fructose, but their fiber and antioxidant content can add to lowering oxidative stress. We would caution against high-sugar fruits, such as pineapple and grapes, in large amounts. It would also be good to avoid dried fruit and fruit juices, since their sugar content tends to be higher and can be an issue, especially for people with diabetes. Fresh fruit is likely the most potent, so try to eat whole fruits. Try to vary the fruits you eat because they all offer different nutrients. Citrus has vitamin C. Berries are abundant in antioxidants. Bananas are rich in potassium.

People with diabetes often tell us their doctors say they cannot eat fruits. But then those same people eat refined breads and cookies because they want something sweet and they're hungry. We would take any fruit over that option, any day of the week. Most often, the fruit is not the problem for people with diabetes; usually everything else in the diet is the culprit.

Overall, fruits and vegetables are great when eaten raw. However, there are some vegetables that are more nutritionally potent when they are cooked. It's hard to remember exactly which vegetables are more potent when cooked, so we try to keep it simple and just tell people to eat as many colors as they can throughout the day: raw, cooked, frozen, whatever. The bottom line is eating more than seven servings per day of fruits and vegetables lowers heart disease risk and has a role in decreasing cancer and all-cause mortality.

Many people feel overwhelmed when they consider that they have to eat seven servings of fruits and vegetables every day. People often ask how to incorporate them into their meals. In the morning, Dr. A often has a banana and two pieces of toast with hummus. She eats fresh bread from the bakery, which has minimal sugar and no preservatives. Then around 10:00 a.m., she eats 20 to 30 baby carrots, usually with hummus again. For lunch, she often eats a huge spinach or kale salad with an abundance of vegetables and seeds. Around 3:00 p.m., she might have an apple. For dinner, she will often eat a bean burrito with steamed broccoli, or a bowl of rice and lentils with that same steamed broccoli or sautéed bok choy. For dessert, an orange (or nothing at all) is enough.

When you think it through, it can be easy to get seven to ten servings of vegetables per day! Bottom line is to try for diversity and remember to eat all of the colorful vegetables—don't limit yourself. For instance, red and yellow peppers are full of phytonutrients. Spinach is full of iron but doesn't provide calcium and may even leach calcium you've just eaten from other sources. Turnip greens, mustard greens, bok choy, and kale, among others, have plenty of calcium, so vary it up and eat all the colorful vegetables, all of the time. (See Consider 2 on the next page.)

CONSIDER 2

✓ When you are thinking about your fruits and vegetables for the day, you don't have to remember what fruit or vegetable has what in it. Just remember to eat a variety of colors. Eat greens, reds, oranges, blues, and purples. Don't get stuck on just one color; you won't get the full benefits.

A Few Words about Kale

Kale has received a lot of press lately as the wonder vegetable, a superfood. It really is an amazing vegetable. It contains an abundance of vitamin A, potassium, and magnesium. It also has iron, calcium, and protein and a bounty of B vitamins, including folate, which helps in brain development. Kale also contains fiber, which is good for lowering cholesterol levels, as well as alpha-linolenic acid (ALA), a precursor to omega-3 fatty acids. ALA also has been shown to decrease the risk of heart disease.[13] Omega-3 fatty acids are important in decreasing inflammation and should be part of the daily diet. Kale also has lutein, which helps to prevent macular degeneration. We try to eat kale at least three times per week. You can choose from three different types of kale: lacinato, green, and red Russian kale. They are all good! Eat them all. Remove the stems from kale (they are difficult to eat, especially raw); you can add finely chopped stems to a soup or broth.

Juices and Shakes

We often hear questions about juices and shakes. Whole fruits and vegetables, rather than juices, are absolutely the best and should be encouraged. In their liquid form, as with juicing, all of the essential fibers are removed from the food. You have nothing to chew on to stimulate your gut enzymes, which are essential for good digestion. When we juice, we get vitamins and lots of sugar without that fiber. When we eat food raw, we get so much more. If you really like to drink juice, drink small amounts and think about pomegranate juice, which has many potent antioxidants.

What about shakes? We do use a heavy-duty blender on occasion. When you use these blenders, the fruits and vegetables are broken down, but the fiber stays inside the drink. That fiber content is good, but probably not as good as the whole food because the fibers are broken up. When you eat the whole food, you have to chew, which activates the digestive enzymes. Whole fiber brings down your cholesterol levels and decreases inflammation. At the end of the day, shakes are good because they are quick and allow an easy way to get in a lot of vegetables at once. Are whole fruits and vegetables even a little better? Sure! Do the best you can. If shakes work, go for it.

ADD BACK #2: Carbohydrates—Legumes and Beans

Carbohydrates (carbs) have gotten a bad rap lately, and we want to give you our two cents about the underappreciated carbohydrate. So many diets tell us to avoid carbohydrates because they are the reason we gain weight. This concept is the foundation for many low-carb or no-carb diets, which often focus on counting carbs to keep weight down. We don't believe in these diets and counting carbs. Without carbs, we lose so many essential nutrients and fiber. Carbs also allow us to feel full. The nutrients in carbohydrates are essential because they provide us with the energy for day-to-day living. They give us our energy to get up and go. People gain weight when they eat carbs, for the most part, because the carbs they are eating are refined and highly processed, not the whole-grain carbohydrates they should be eating. When you eat whole-grain carbs, your body will tell you when to stop eating. You will feel full, content, and energetic.

Let's talk about chemistry a bit. Carbohydrates can be broken into complex carbohydrates and simple carbohydrates. The simple carbs are mostly sugars. They are good for short bursts of energy but have no lasting effect. The more complex the structure of a carbohydrate, the longer it takes to break it down, which causes less rise in blood glucose (blood sugar) levels. This is the concept of the glycemic index. Foods that have a low glycemic index are more complex in structure—more whole-grain—and take longer to break down and, thus, raise your blood glucose to only a low level. Those foods high on the glycemic index, such as candy, chips, cookies, and other processed foods, are simple sugars and break down easily. Because low-glycemic index foods take longer to break down, they bring about a feeling of satiety faster than high-glycemic foods and with less drastic boosts in blood sugar levels.

It is not only a food's ranking on the glycemic index that's important, though. Food in its natural form provides a lot of fiber. Beans are carbohydrates but are full of fiber and water, so they take longer to break down. Because they take time to break down, they don't cause the quick highs and lows that foods high in simple sugars, such as refined breads and sodas, can cause; they steadily break down over time. These complex carbohydrates give us a measured amount of energy at all times. It gets a little confusing when we look at pasta. Pasta is a low-glycemic food, which is good, but it has minimal fiber. On the other hand, it is better than eating candy and cookies, which have a high glycemic index without any fiber and, therefore, are processed moderately quickly. Pasta is good and filling but doesn't have the fiber we need.

While fruits are considered simple carbohydrates because they are primarily sugar, but they are good for us because they also provide us with fiber and nutrients. As you can see, not all simple carbohydrates are a problem. It is what we do to the foods, the processing, that is problematic. When we process them, they become simple, their glycemic index increases, and they lose their fiber: two negatives. Studies show that increased fiber is associated with decreased heart disease.[14] Studies also show that whole grains are better than simple or refined grains.[15]

The foundational complex carbohydrates are legumes, which come from plants. They have a low glycemic index and are high in fiber. (See figure 2 on the next page.) Examples of legumes are alfalfa, clover, lentils, peas (green peas and chickpeas), beans, carob, soybeans, peanuts, and tamarind. Beans of any kind are excellent food choices. Consider kidney beans, black beans, navy beans, and pinto beans; they are all amazing! There are so many vital ingredients in these legumes. They are rich in protein and high in potassium. Many contain a significant amount of magnesium and iron. Some legumes also provide a little calcium, but not a significant amount.

Legumes also contain resistant starches. When resistant starches reach the colon, they ferment and form short-chain fatty acids, such as butyrate. Butyrate is a short chain fatty acid, and its production appears to be important in maintaining colonic health and lowering

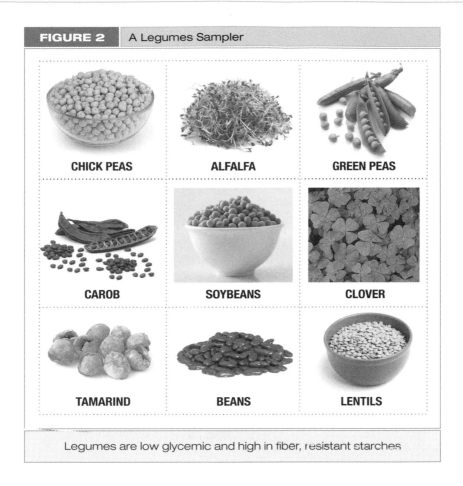

FIGURE 2 | A Legumes Sampler

CHICK PEAS	ALFALFA	GREEN PEAS
CAROB	SOYBEANS	CLOVER
TAMARIND	BEANS	LENTILS

Legumes are low glycemic and high in fiber, resistant starches

our risk of chronic illness. Research suggests that butyrate also is vital in lowering insulin resistance, risk of stroke, and high cholesterol. It also appears related to a diminished risk of cancer.[16] Legumes are truly amazing foods!

Caloric Density

Another way to look at foods is based on their caloric density. Jeff Novick at the McDougall Center in Santa Rosa, California, is a huge proponent of this approach to food. Think of caloric density as the amount of calories per ounce of food. Water and fiber in food will lower its calorie density, while fat and oil increase it. Studies show that overall, people eat about the same amount of food every day, but if you eat, say, half a pound of calorie-dense food such as glazed donuts, you'll take in many more calories than if you eat half a pound of lettuce, which has very little calorie density.

We also need water and fiber in foods to increase satiety. Consider that chili is high in caloric density, but if you add vegetables to chili, its density will be less because vegetables are full of fiber and water. Studies show that people who eat lower caloric-density foods can eat more food by weight and still take in fewer calories than those who eat high-fat, high-caloric-density foods.[17] In other words, you don't have to restrict your portions if you eat foods that are low in calories. You will also feel full because you haven't restricted your portions. The Centers for Disease Control (CDC) points out that people who eat lower caloric-density foods can consume fewer calories without changing how much they eat.[18] Many studies show that when people eat foods with low caloric density, they lose weight without changing the amount they eat, and they feel satiated.[19,20] (See Consider 3 below and figure 3 on the next page.)

CONSIDER 3

 If you eat low-calorie-dense foods, you don't have to restrict your portions. You can take in the same amount of food and maybe even more, but with that, you will take in fewer calories and still feel full.

Then, we can eat an abundance of beans, lentils, and chickpeas in our diets. They are our main protein source, so we eat them at least once every day—usually a spinach salad for lunch with beans on top. You can put loads of vegetables and beans in the salad and feel full without adding croutons or French dressing (which is processed). Instead, make a hummus-based dressing, or use balsamic vinegar to flavor the salad. We find that the beans themselves are quite flavorful and often carry the taste of the salad.

Oatmeal also is good for you, but adding bananas and raspberries makes it even better because it lowers caloric density while adding the multiple benefits of the fruits. Eating bread is okay, but adding hummus and an abundance of raw green vegetables makes it delicious, and the vegetables lower the caloric density. A diet with these qualities is filling and provides the essential nutrients required in daily living

FIGURE 3	Examples of Low Density and High Density Meals

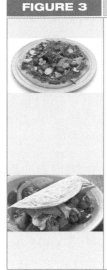

Low Calorie Density Meal (GOOD)

- 12 oz water
- Kale salad with hummus
- Veggie pizza without cheese
- Or bowl of rice and beans with sprouts, onions, tomatoes and spinach
- Low calorie density snack: raw veggies and hummus

High Calorie Density Meal (NOT GOOD)

- Juice
- Beef taco with shredded cheese, sour cream
- Grilled chicken, beans, sour cream in burrito
- High calorie dense snack: granola bar or cheese stick

without unnecessary toxins. Adding those raw veggies and fruits will make all the difference in reaching your wellness goals.

Our intention is to not restrict your portions, within reason. If you eat the right foods all of the time, you won't have to weigh yourself every day or count points or calories. Throw away all of that nonsense! We want you to think about eating whole grains and plant-based proteins, such as legumes. We try to teach our patients how much of our lifestyle is correctable with diet. Learning to eat foods we aren't used to, or may not like, is difficult. We often tell our children that they don't have to like everything they eat; they just have to eat it. Our hope is that once they have tried eating enough healthier foods, they too will learn to love them.

Change is hard work. Eating healthy and exercising is hard work. For some, it will initially seem like an impossible task. People find it inconceivable to drink water in the morning with oatmeal and fruit, instead of coffee with cream and sugar and two pieces of buttered toast or processed cereals. People say to us that they don't care to change. They want to eat their meat and take their cholesterol medications too. Does that work? Unfortunately, it doesn't. Our cholesterol numbers might be better, but our bodies are still inflamed, overweight, and overtired. The body is still on fire. It all has to change.

With that in mind, do the best you can. We drink caffeine. We just drink caffeinated teas without dairy. We break down occasionally and snack, but we often feel tired and uncomfortable when we do. We don't exercise every day. We don't sleep as much as we would like. Life happens. You do the best you can, but every bit of change helps. You will find, though, that your energy is so much better with these changes. You won't have the highs and lows in energy based on the foods you eat because the food will be processed slowly in your system.

Is This a Diet? The Plant-Based Lifestyle

S o does a plant-based lifestyle work? Absolutely. In Dean Ornish's early work, he showed that with lifestyle modification, we can reverse heart disease. In his original work published in 1996, he directed 48 individuals with moderate to severe coronary artery disease to make lifestyle changes. They were put on a 10 percent fat vegetarian diet, encouraged to do moderate aerobic exercise, and were given stress management training and smoking cessation counseling. Over one year (and more impressively over five years), plaque regression was noted in the treatment group and progression of atherosclerotic disease was noted in the control group.[21] The lifestyle changes worked! (See Consider 4.)

CONSIDER 4

✔ Think about the power of having a tool that acts like a medication without being one. These lifestyle changes not only stabilize plaque but may have the power to cause plaque regression.

In 1995, an assessment of the Mediterranean diet, featuring an abundance of vegetables, fruit, and fiber, suggested that following the diet reduces heart disease risk. Further, researchers suggested that dairy intake is related to higher heart disease risk. Researchers in this trial also stated that the connection between higher dairy intake and lowering fracture rate is limited.[22] In another trial from 2002, it was noted that the optimal diet for lowering risk of coronary artery disease was a diet with non-hydrogenated fats, whole grains, and an abundance of fruits and vegetables.[23]

Many trials have examined the relationships between vegetables and fruit and heart disease and have shown an inverse relationship between increased consumption of fruits and vegetables and decreased risk of heart disease. The Lyons Diet study showed that eating more fruits and vegetables, and the alpha-linolenic acid (ALA) found in the Mediterranean diet, reduced the incidence of myocardial infarctions (heart attacks) and mortality, compared with a regular low-fat diet in patients with known heart disease.[24] Many more trials show the role of fruits and vegetables in lowering blood pressure.[25]

Regarding whole grains, the Iowa Women's Health Study showed that when people ate more whole grains, they suffered fewer cardiovascular events.[26] In the Nurses' Health Study, a 25 percent decrease in cardiovascular events was noted in women who ate more than three servings of whole grains per day versus those who ate less than one serving per day![27]

Two important studies highlight the benefits of a plant-based diet compared to the standard Western diet. In the Nurses' Health Study, nurses were given either a whole-grain, plant-based diet or the standard Western diet, which is abundant in meat and processed meats, French fries, and sweets.[28] There was a 25 percent risk reduction in eating the whole-grain, plant-based diet compared to the standard Western diet. Similar results were also noted in the Health Professionals Follow-Up Study.[29]

There were also noncardiovascular benefits to the Mediterranean diet. In the Nurses' Health Study, women who adopted this diet were found to have longer telomeres, which, if you recall, are associated with longevity![30] This data is compelling. It works. The data shows that a plant-based lifestyle is a healthier option than the alternative.

A Word on Fermented Foods

Fermentation is the process of converting sugars to acids, gases, or alcohol. It occurs in the presence of bacteria and yeast and in our muscles when they are oxygen-depleted and lactic acid builds up. Fermentation creates many useful bacteria and enhances their nutritional effects with increased numbers of vitamins and omega-3 fatty acids. We view eating fermented foods as opportunities to naturally nourish the gut. They are natural probiotics. Examples of these fermented foods are kimchi (pickled vegetables from Korea), sauerkraut (fermented cabbage), kombucha (fermented tea), miso (fermented soy paste), and tempeh (fermented soybeans). These are fabulous foods that we try to include in our diets a few times a week. You don't have to make them yourself; we buy jars of sauerkraut and kimchi and eat them with pita bread and hummus. We cook with tempeh and eat miso soup. All good options to add the natural bacteria back into our bodies!

So Why Not Go on a Diet? Because They Don't Work

Research shows that approximately two-thirds of people who go on a specific weight-loss diet will fail to keep off the weight. A study published in *American Psychologist* reviewed 31 diet plans and their success rates. Researchers found that after reaching their goal weights, one-third to two-thirds of the dieters regained not only the weight lost on the diet, but most gained even more weight than they had initially lost.[31] The authors of that study recognized that these percentages may be underestimating the actual incidence of weight regain, due to the way the follow-up programs were conducted. In eight of the studies, approximately 50 percent of the dieters did not participate in the follow-up surveys, and in many other studies, the follow-up was done remotely (not in person), with no true measurements of weight by an independent party. So people probably gained more weight than was recorded.

Most of us are not happy with failures in our lives, so many people may not have responded honestly to the remote survey as the pounds started creeping back. But it may not be a personal failure that they failed to keep off the weight; people simply are not taught how to eat.

The key is to learn how to substitute whole, healthy foods that can then become your favorite foods. We hope to help you on this journey—not to give you a short-term diet but, rather, to help you change your way of life.

For about the last 60 years in America, we've celebrated special occasions with sodas, sweet desserts, cakes, pies, candies, and ice cream. As these foods have become readily available, many people have come to eat those high-calorie, nutrient-deficient foods every single day. But regularly consuming what used to be special-occasion, highly caloric treats is making us overweight and obese. Many people drink sodas or other sweetened drinks all day long, every day of the week. Add that to fast food, donuts, other pastries and desserts, ice cream, and other processed foods, and we are eating way too much processed sweeteners and flours, which are nutrient-poor, high-calorie foods.

Specific diets can be very difficult to maintain in the real world. Most diet plans do not address food addictions, the dangers of processed sweeteners, the necessity of fruits and vegetables, hydration, or a proper balance of complex carbohydrates, healthy proteins, and fats. People are told to stop eating this and stop eating that, but they're not told what to eat instead. Many physicians say people cannot change and that we, as physicians, always recommend dietary changes, but most people do not comply. We believe that people don't comply because they haven't been taught how to eat. People need guidance and support. We think if people were presented the information in a positive way, we would see more people adopting healthier lifestyles.

There are also the diets that restrict one macronutrient: either protein, fat, or carbohydrate. Many popular restrictive diets suggest restricting carbohydrates. You can lose a lot of weight quickly on a low-carbohydrate, high-protein, high-fat diet. Recent studies show minimal difference in weight loss between a low-carb and low-fat diet.[32]

Low-carb diets put the body into a state of ketosis, which is known to accelerate fat loss, and this lures many people into trying it. For people who already enjoy eating high-protein, fatty foods, such as bacon, steak, cheese, and hamburgers, this sounds like the perfect answer. Eliminate or severely restrict carbohydrates and eat all the steak and bacon you can! Portion control is often not specified in these plans, so eating large portions may be encouraged. Some people may actually see elevated cholesterol levels on a high-fat, high-protein diet, even though they may be losing weight. *Do you know how many stents we have put into patients who eat like this?*

Ketosis is the result of the body burning fat for energy instead of burning the body's normal fuel, complex carbohydrates. People can actually test their urine to see if they are in ketosis. Consuming large amounts of animal protein may be hard on the kidneys to begin with, and a prolonged state of ketosis might possibly stress the kidneys even more. This can be particularly difficult and potentially dangerous for those who are diabetic, pregnant, or have been diagnosed with kidney disease.[33]

In these types of diets, the fact that the body needs the complex carbohydrates found in fresh fruits and vegetables is ignored. Complex carbohydrates normally provide fuel for the body and offer a huge variety of complex micronutrients and vitamins that can be lacking in most fats and proteins. Typically, once weight loss has been achieved, the dieter will return to his or her previous eating habits with no knowledge of portion control or balanced nutrition. Again, weight gain most likely will occur.

Other diet plans suggest simply either counting calories or counting carbohydrates or both. There are many new computer and smartphone apps that will track your consumption of calories and carbohydrates each day. These high-tech applications attempt to overcome the drudgery and complexity of all that counting. People don't understand that keeping track of only calories or carbohydrates does not show you the nutritional quality of those calories. Simply reducing calories is not the answer. People also feel hungry all of the time when they limit calories. Recall, legumes and beans cause butyrate production, which triggers leptin and tells us we are full. Counting carbs and cutting calories make us feel hungry and unsatisfied. Ironically, counting is not necessary when one is consuming a whole-food diet of predominantly fresh vegetables, legumes (dried beans and lentils), fruits, and whole grains.

Bottom Line: Overeating, drinking sodas (sweetened or artificially sweetened), dehydration, eating predominantly packaged foods, and lack of exercise are major causes of most obesity in America today. Diets do not work, but lifestyle changes do. Eating healthy, whole, fresh foods; avoiding packaged foods; staying hydrated; and exercising regularly create the formula for achieving and maintaining a healthy weight. It sounds difficult, but you can begin simply by making small changes—drink a glass of water in the morning, go for a walk, buy some fresh vegetables and fruits, and read the labels on any packaged foods you may want to buy. This is your life—choose health!

Many people think it is too expensive to eat healthy whole foods, but it really isn't; it just takes a little bit of planning. Brown rice, lentils, quinoa, and dried beans are some of the least expensive foods available. They offer plenty of nutrients, fiber, vitamins, and minerals. Cooked dry beans are another excellent source of fiber and protein.

Shopping for fresh local vegetables and fruits at farmer's markets and buying frozen vegetables and fruits at the grocery store are other effective ways to minimize your costs for healthy food options. Remember to always read the labels on packaged foods to ensure there have been no added sweeteners or other unhealthy ingredients. Be sure the only ingredient is the actual fruit or vegetable.

YOUR PRESCRIPTION

EAT SMART

The right food choices can make a big difference in your health.

1. Try to get five to seven servings of fruits and vegetables per day. Eat more vegetables than fruit.

2. Eat lots of colorful vegetables every day.

3. Learn to eat beans and lentils every day.

4. Don't be afraid of carbs. Eat whole grains. You will feel great, and weight loss will be a side effect.

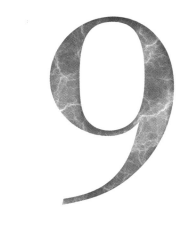

Oil Change

NUTS, SEEDS, AND AVOCADO

What is the deal with fats and oils?

here is so much conversation in the media about fat. Is it good, bad, or ugly?! In order to answer that question, we need to explain what fat is and what it does. Fats can be broken down into saturated fats and unsaturated fats. Unsaturated fats are further broken down into monounsaturated fats (MUFAs) and polyunsaturated fats (PUFAs). PUFAs are further broken down into the essential fatty acids (EFAs): omega-3 and omega-6 fatty acids. Let's go through this in more detail now. (See figure 1 on the next page.)

Saturated Fats

aturated fats are solid at room temperature. They are very stable and have a long shelf life. The most common saturated fats are found in butter and other animal fats, such as milk, cheese, and meat. Saturated fats are found in both animal and plant products. Examples of plant substances that have saturated fats are coconut oil, palm oil, palm kernel oil, cocoa butter, and avocado. The general feeling is that saturated fats should be avoided because they will increase risk of cardiovascular disease. In 1908, rabbits were given a diet high in cholesterol and saturated fats, and their atherosclerosis (hardening of the arteries) increased.[1] In the 1950s, studies showed that a diet rich in saturated fats and cholesterol was associated with higher cholesterol levels in humans.[2] Epidemiologic studies performed around that time also showed that higher cholesterol predicted one's risk of coronary heart disease.[3] This led to the diet-heart hypothesis, which postulated that eating saturated fats and cholesterol can lead to heart disease.[4] Later studies continue to show that too much saturated fat is bad for the heart.[5, 6] Therefore, there should be no dispute in our minds about whether saturated fat is good or bad. Reducing saturated fat is recommended in all cardiovascular prevention guidelines.[7] Saturated fat is not good for us.

But wait . . . some of you might be wondering about the PURE trial, which came out recently, that said that saturated fat is not the enemy.[8] It is actually carbohydrate, and we just told you that saturated fats are bad. As we point out in our editorial response to the PURE trial, it is not that saturated fat is good and carbohydrate is bad, but rather that saturated fat is bad and simple, refined carbohydrates are worse.[9,10] The

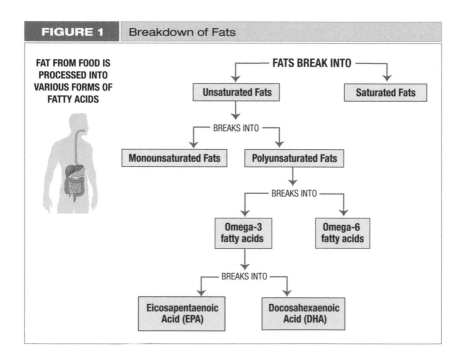

FIGURE 1   Breakdown of Fats

FAT FROM FOOD IS PROCESSED INTO VARIOUS FORMS OF FATTY ACIDS

FATS BREAK INTO

Unsaturated Fats

Saturated Fats

BREAKS INTO

Monounsaturated Fats

Polyunsaturated Fats

BREAKS INTO

Omega-3 fatty acids

Omega-6 fatty acids

BREAKS INTO

Eicosapentaenoic Acid (EPA)

Docosahexaenoic Acid (DHA)

bottom line: the goal should be to continue to avoid saturated fats and refined carbohydrates.

But here is the dilemma. Saturated fats are very useful for the food industry because they have a long shelf life. Foods made with lard and other animal fats last longer. When saturated fats were thought to be unhealthy, food producers had to reconsider how foods were being prepared. Interest shifted to unsaturated fats.

The Shift to Polyunsaturated Fats

W hen saturated fats fell out of vogue, food producers started looking at unsaturated fats as an alternative. We mentioned that unsaturated fats are broken into PUFAs and MUFAs. PUFAs are fats that are liquid at room temperature, such as vegetable oils (corn oil), but they also can be found in sources such as whole grains, nuts, and seeds. When we extract the oils from corn (corn oil), seeds, and other vegetables, we are extracting pure fat. All of the beneficial fiber is removed, as well as many of the other nutrients found in the whole food. Most processed oils are used in packaged or processed foods and for cooking, in salad dressings, and in dips. Studies have shown that when saturated fat is exchanged for PUFAs, there is reduced cardiovascular risk.[11] The problem with this substitution is that PUFAs have a poor shelf life, which is a problem for food manufacturers. This led to the advent of the worst fat in our society—*and we created it*: trans fat (see page 97). First, we have to break down what is in polyunsaturated fats. PUFAs can be broken into omega-3 and omega-6 fatty acids.

Omega-3 Fatty Acids

O mega-3 fatty acids have been studied extensively, mostly from marine sources. Omega-3 fatty acids are important for reducing triglycerides (fat in the blood). Recent studies of highly concentrated omega-3 fatty acids in pill form (marketed as icosapent ethyl) show that they can reduce the risk of a cardiovascular event in people with elevated triglycerides along with either cardiovascular disease or diabetes plus another risk factor.[12]

Omega-3 fatty acids may also lower your risk of abnormal heart rhythms,[13] aid in blood thinning, and may help to improve dilation

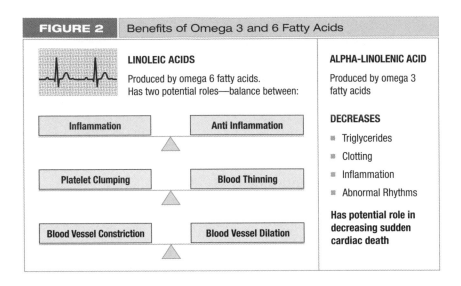

FIGURE 2 | Benefits of Omega 3 and 6 Fatty Acids

LINOLEIC ACIDS
Produced by omega 6 fatty acids.
Has two potential roles—balance between:

| Inflammation | Anti Inflammation |

| Platelet Clumping | Blood Thinning |

| Blood Vessel Constriction | Blood Vessel Dilation |

ALPHA-LINOLENIC ACID
Produced by omega 3 fatty acids

DECREASES
- Triglycerides
- Clotting
- Inflammation
- Abnormal Rhythms

Has potential role in decreasing sudden cardiac death

of blood vessels.[14] It's been shown that people who consume two or more servings of fish per week have an increased lifespan.[15] In studies, these improvements in lifespan were noted with marine omega-3 fatty acids and were most notable when intake was as high as 30 percent of calories. Omega-3 fatty acids are comprised of eicosapentaenoic acid (EPA) and docosahexaenoic acid (DHA), which have been shown to be key factors in decreasing coronary heart disease.[3] Alpha-linolenic acid (ALA) is an omega-3 fatty acid found in plant sources, such as flaxseed, canola oil, and soybean oil, and can be converted to EPA and DHA in the body. However, there is some debate about how effective plant-based sources of omega-3 fatty acids are relative to marine sources, because there is some inefficiency in the conversion of plant-based sources of omega-3 fatty acids to DHA and EPA. However, ALA has been shown to improve cardiovascular outcomes and decrease heart disease.[16,17] (See figure 2.)

Omega-6 Fatty Acids

Besides omega-3 fatty acids, there is much discussion about omega-6 fatty acids. You'll recall that unsaturated fats can be divided into omega-3 and omega-6 fatty acids. Many people feel that omega-3 fatty acids are the "good" fatty acids and omega-6 fatty acids are the "bad" ones. However, is that really true? The main omega-6 fatty acid is linoleic acid (different from the alpha-linolenic acid made by omega-3 fatty acids). Linoleic acid is found in foods such as corn, soy, sunflower, and safflower. When linoleic acid is ingested, it breaks down into eicosanoids, some of which promote inflammation, platelet aggregation (potential for plaque formation), and tightening of the blood vessels, and some that have the opposite effect and promote anti-inflammation, decrease platelet aggregation, and dilate blood vessels. We are not entirely clear of the percentages of the eicosanoid that each food creates or what the optimal balance in our bodies is. (See figure 2.)

We typically think of inflammation, platelet aggregation, and tightening of the blood vessels as bad things, but the body certainly needs some omega-6 fats from the diet for proper blood clotting and appropriate inflammation to heal the body's injuries. If we didn't clot, we could bleed out when we cut ourselves or fall and skin a knee! Remember that inflammation is a normal response to a bodily insult. It is the body's response to stress. That stress triggers the body to heal and respond to the attack. However, with continuous stress on the body, the body becomes imbalanced, and that triggers uncontrolled inflammation. Then, it can be seen that we need some amounts of both omega-3 and omega-6 fatty acids. The right balance, however, is not so clear.

Why don't we know what the right balance of omega-3 and omega-6 acids is? The problem is that human trials of omega-6 fatty acids are imperfect. We have some data showing that higher doses of omega-6 fatty acids can cause oxidation (not good) of LDL and may promote inflammation.[18] Other studies suggest that all PUFAs (omega-3 and omega-6 fatty acids both) are associated with narrowing of blood vessels.[19] In contrast, some studies suggest an LDL-lowering effect of omega-6 fatty acids when omega-6 PUFAs were substituted for saturated fats.[20] This, however, may not be because omega-6 PUFAs are good in isolation but that they are better than saturated fats.

Unfortunately, there are no clinical trials that specifically look at outcomes from adding omega-6 fatty acids to the diet and assessing outcomes. Many observational studies show either a small benefit from additional omega-6 fatty acids or no benefit at all.[21] However, two studies show that the omega-6 fatty acid, Linolenic acid, was associated with decreased heart disease.[22] Overall, the American Heart Association now suggests that 5 to 10 percent of our diets should be omega-6 fatty acids, which may bring about a decrease in coronary heart disease.[23]

How much omega-6 fatty acid we should include in our diets and what ratio of omega-3 to omega-6 to consume continues to be debated. Likely, we should attain a balance in our diets between the two or consume more omega-3 fatty acids than omega-6 fatty acids. Currently, however, the average American diet has 14 to 25 times more omega-6 than omega-3.[24] The Mediterranean diet appears to have much a better balance of omega-3 to omega-6 and has been shown to improve health outcomes. All types of fatty acids appear to have a beneficial role to some degree, but we are likely getting too much omega-6 fatty acid in our diets. Therefore, a ratio of 1:1 or 2:1 of omega-6 to omega-3 fats would provide the proper balance for optimal health, allowing the body to clot and heal when injured, but also controlling inflammation and clotting when we are not injured.

So what does that mean in terms of the foods we should eat? (See figure 3.) When we look at oils, the ratio of omega-6 to omega-3 fatty acids is highest in corn oil (48:1), followed by sunflower oil (13:1), and then olive oil (13:1). (Important: olive oil is 72 percent monounsaturated fat and the remainder is polyunsaturated fat). Vegetable and soybean oils follow at 9:1 and 8:1 respectively (courtesy of Jeff Novick from TrueNorth Health Center). Canola oil (rapeseed oil) has a ratio of about 2:1. Flaxseed oil is probably the healthiest oil, with little saturated fat, a large proportion of polyunsaturated fat, and a good ratio of omega-6 to omega-3 fatty acids. Of note, however, is that flaxseed oil cannot be used to cook with, because it is potentially harmful when warmed. (See Consider 1.)

CONSIDER 1

☑ Flaxseed oil has a good ratio of omega-3 to omega-6 fatty acids, but do not use it for cooking. Heating it makes it potentially harmful to the body.

- You can add flaxseed oil to a smoothie.

- You can also add flaxseeds to foods after they have been cooked.

- You can add ground flaxseeds into your oatmeal after it is cooked, or add them to a cereal or smoothie.

- Seeds should be ground; otherwise the seeds will often pass through the body unprocessed and not be beneficial.

- It is okay to bake with flaxseed meal; think about using it in bread, cakes, and muffins.

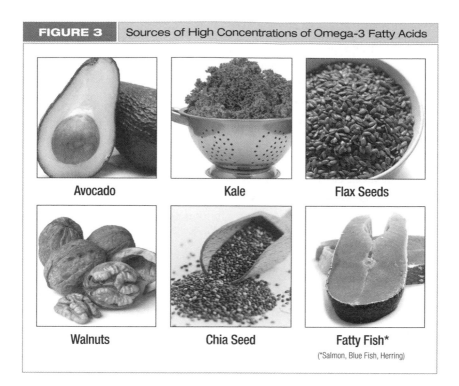

FIGURE 3 | Sources of High Concentrations of Omega-3 Fatty Acids

Avocado   Kale   Flax Seeds

Walnuts   Chia Seed   Fatty Fish*
(*Salmon, Blue Fish, Herring)

Trans Fats

H istorically speaking, the benefits of PUFAs in decreasing heart disease were compelling and well touted, but the food industry struggled because of their poor shelf life. As a result, manufacturers began hydrogenating these oils to make them easier to use and longer lasting. This began the advent of trans fats. It was easy for manufacturers to use trans fats because they were not saturated fats, which had become unpopular due to their potential cardiovascular effects. What's more, trans fats were polyunsaturated fats, so they were considered healthy, and when they were hydrogenated, they had the added benefit of a longer shelf life. Without realizing it, however, manufacturers added highly toxic oils back into our foods that were actually more toxic to our hearts than saturated fats.

Controlled studies have shown that trans fats increase LDL and lower HDL cholesterol, compared to non-hydrogenated unsaturated fatty acids.[25] They also increase lipoprotein[a] (a pro-inflammatory marker) and triglycerides and may reduce the blood vessel's ability to dilate.[26,27]

Trans fats also increase our risk of diabetes.[28] Over the years, clinical trials have become better; they're larger and more randomized and show the negative impact of trans fats on the risk of coronary heart disease.[29] The Nurses' Health Study looked at 80,082 women and found that higher trans fats (and, to a smaller extent, saturated fats) were associated with higher risk of heart disease compared to a diet containing polyunsaturated non-hydrogenated fats.[30]

During the trans fat years, people started looking at the Mediterranean diet more closely. Studies began showing that the Mediterranean diet was linked to lower cardiovascular mortality. Analysis of food oils used in this diet led to the focus on olive oil as the "golden oil" and targeted the abundance of MUFAs and PUFAs in the oil. Olive oil is 72 percent monounsaturated fat. The remainder is linoleic acid, which, as you may recall, is an omega-6 polyunsaturated fat. MUFAs have been shown to lower triglycerides and LDL levels and elevate HDL compared to saturated fats. In some studies, they have been shown to improve cardiovascular outcomes, ease oxidative stress, and improve diabetes control.[31] Olive oil is also rich in polyphenols, which are believed to decrease oxidative stresses on the cells (reduce cell damage).[32]

To date, olive oil has enjoyed the spotlight as the oil used in the Mediterranean diet and, therefore, has been purported as the oil that can improve heart health. People often will add olive oil to their foods because of its cardiovascular benefits, above and beyond their normal food requirements. Many of our patients explain that they are eating olive oil because it is good for the heart. But is that the right thing to do? **The big question:** Is olive oil or any oil actually good for us by itself? Or is it just better than the alternatives—saturated and trans fats?

A study in 1995 was performed on African green monkeys.[33] They were fed three different diets: one high in monounsaturated fats, one high in polyunsaturated fats, and one high in saturated fats. LDL cholesterol levels (bad cholesterol) were fairly similar in the monkeys on the mono- and polyunsaturated diets, which were lower than the group eating the saturated fat diet. HDL cholesterol levels (good cholesterol—we want this high) was similar between the groups eating saturated fat and monounsaturated fats and lowest in the group eating polyunsaturated fats. When you look at coronary artery disease in these monkeys, though, regardless of the type of fat in their diet, they all developed atherosclerosis—clogging of the arteries. The amount of disease was similar between the groups eating monounsaturated and saturated fats. So, if all groups, despite the food being primarily full of mono- or polyunsaturated or saturated fats, developed heart disease, is oil ever really a good thing?

Interestingly, atherosclerotic plaque was lowest in the group eating polyunsaturated fats, which actually had the lowest levels of that good HDL cholesterol. This was likely due to changes in LDL particle composition and higher amount of omega-3 fatty acids. Jeff Novick, when he was at the Pritikin Center, also noted a University of Crete study.[34] In that study, researchers looked retrospectively at people with heart disease and those who were heart-healthy and found that those who had heart disease had a diet higher in olive oil and fats compared to those who did not. It was more information supporting the notion that oil of any type causes heart plaque.

More information was found when looking at the work of Dr. A's former mentors, Robert Vogel, MD, and colleagues at the University of Maryland. Physicians Vogel, Coretti, and Plotnick did a study in which they looked at dilatation of blood vessels by giving subjects food that emphasized different portions of the Mediterranean diet (olive oil, canola oil, and salmon).[35] They found that individuals who received canola oil or salmon actually had more open blood vessels compared to the other groups. On the other hand, olive oil caused a reduction in the opening of the blood vessels. In their conclusion, they noted that a diet full of antioxidant-rich foods, such as fruits, vegetables, fish, vinegar, and canola oils, are the important parts of the Mediterranean diet, rather than olive oil. Here again, the findings point out that perhaps olive oil is not the wonder food that it has been purported to be. (See Consider 2.)

CONSIDER 2

☑ Olive oil is *not* the wonder oil. There is no oil that is good for us. Having no oil is better than any of the oils. All oils have the ability to cause heart plaque.

All three classes of fatty acids (saturated fats, monounsaturated fats, and polyunsaturated fats) increase HDL when they replace complex carbohydrates in the diet. This increase is slightly higher in monounsaturated fats than with saturated fats. Monounsaturated fats are believed to lower cholesterol more than saturated fats when replacing saturated fats on a pound-per-pound basis. As such, it is not that these oils were thought to be healthy; they were just seen as better than the saturated fats they were replacing. When the components of the Mediterranean diet were carefully analyzed, a few important points were realized. (See Consider 3.)

CONSIDER 3

✓ When the components of the Mediterranean diet were analyzed three main points were derived.

1. Consumption of fruits, vegetables, and legumes decreased mortality; meaning the more of them you eat, the less likely you are to die.

2. With respect to dairy and meat, a positive association was found between consumption and mortality, so the more consumption, the larger the mortality risk.

3. While the Mediterranean diet has an emphasis on olive oil, it is not clear that olive oil is good for you.

Calorie Density of Oils

Caloric density refers to the calories per gram or pound of a substance. Oils, pound per pound, are some of the most calorie-dense substances, and one tablespoon of oil typically provides 14 grams of fat (just over 120 calories, all from fat)! People are always surprised by how much fat is in oil. Think about this when you are sprinkling oil and vinegar on your salad.

Avocado

Let's talk about the avocado for a moment because it has come under a great deal of scrutiny. Avocados are highly potent fruits. They are full of potassium, magnesium, iron, B vitamins, and vitamins C and E. They possess the carotenoid lutein, which is good for our eyes, and folate, which is crucial for cell repair. Avocados are high poly- and monounsaturated fats. But they also contain saturated fat and are calorie-dense fruits.

Overall, an avocado is a filling and primarily healthy food. But eating too many can cause weight gain and potentially increase cholesterol. For people with known heart disease or multiple risk factors, avocado intake should probably be restricted. However, for many, an avocado is a filling, nutrient-rich option to add to a plant-based, whole-grain diet.

A Word on Coconut Oil

T o finish the historical assessment of oil, we need to talk about coconut and palm oils. After trans fats were banned, the food industry started looking for other oils that were not animal-based and had a long shelf life. The search for so-called good fats was becoming something of a journey. First, saturated fats were used in abundance, and then their negative effects were discovered. PUFAs were felt to be good but had poor shelf life. We found later that hydrogenating PUFAs to make trans fats was actually worse. People shifted to non-hydrogenated PUFAs and MUFAs.

Individuals in the food industry started asking if there were any other options. They continued to look for cheap, palatable oils with a long shelf life. This brought attention to coconut and palm kernel oil, which are plant-based oils that are high in saturated fats. For instance, coconut oil is 90 percent saturated. The remainder is a small amount of unsaturated fat, primarily omega-6 fatty acids.

What do we know about coconut oil? Not much, really. We know from early studies that saturated fats increase our risk of cardiovascular mortality and that the hydrogenated forms of coconut oils that were popular in the 1980s were extremely harmful. We learned from the monkey studies that all oils cause atherosclerotic disease. Coconut oil also doesn't have a good ratio of omega-3s to omega-6s, so it appears to be pro-inflammatory. Is there more to it, though? Why has it become popular?

Coconut oil is different from other saturated fats because it is primarily made of medium-chain triglycerides (lauric acid). There is some preliminary data on its role in preventing Alzheimer's disease. One trial from 2009 looked at 20 women ages 20 to 40 years.[37] They were asked to eat a low-calorie diet and walk 50 minutes every day. They were given 30 milliliters of soybean oil or coconut oil. The coconut oil group was noted to have slightly higher HDL levels (49 gm/dL versus 45 gm/dL) and a slightly better ratio of LDL cholesterol to HDL cholesterol.

This difference was quite small, though. There was also an association regarding weight loss in the coconut oil group.

Because coconut oil is made of medium-chain fatty acids instead of long-chain fatty acids like most other fats, some scientists believe it is not stored in the body as fat deposits. It may even be associated with fat burning. It may allow for more efficient processing of fat. Data from studies performed on mice show that those who were given medium-chain fatty acids had less muscle fatigue. So does coconut oil deserve the hype it has received? Unfortunately, very little is known about this oil, and we would suggest it be used with caution. An oil that is 90 percent saturated fat concerns us. We know that in the African monkeys studies, plaque formed in all the monkeys' blood vessels regardless of the type of oil they were given. For us, it is not a recommended oil. But it is really good as a hair conditioner!

What About Nuts?

Nuts have become very popular lately as heart-healthy foods. Nuts are packed with unsaturated fats, both mono- and polyunsaturated fats. Then, because they have PUFAs, they also are rich in omega-3 and omega-6 fatty acids. Nuts also have fiber, which helps lower our cholesterol and makes us feel full. They also contain vitamin E, which may play a role in reducing heart plaque development. Importantly, nuts have plant sterols, which help to lower cholesterol. They are known to also decrease oxidative stress, and they are rich in L-arginine, which may help with dilatation of the blood vessels and make them less prone to clogs.[37,38] (See figure 3 on page 97 and Consider 4 below.)

CONSIDER 4

✓ Nuts are filled with unsaturated fats. They have fiber and plant sterols that lower cholesterol, decrease oxidative stress, and dilate our blood vessels. Overall, nuts are a good part of our diets, in moderation.

It is important to remember that nuts are high in caloric density, so they should not be eaten in great numbers and not regularly. While nuts were also part of the Mediterranean diet, they were not a large enough portion of the diet to justify high intakes.

There is a lot of interesting data on nuts. The Adventist Health Study is one that showed people who ate nuts more than four times per week had fewer cardiovascular events compared to those who consumed less than one serving per week.[39] Serving size was about one ounce, two to five times per week. In another study, when a small group of men following a restricted diet and fairly equivalent fats and calories shifted 20 percent of their fats and calories to come from walnuts, their total cholesterol dropped, as well as both their LDL and HDL cholesterol levels.[40] In the Nurses' Health Study, there also appeared to be a beneficial effect to eating nuts in terms of decreasing heart disease.[41] But this is observational data, and while the nurses who ate nuts had less heart disease, those nurses also exercised more, ate less meat, were leaner, and smoked less. (See Consider 5.)

CONSIDER 5

✓ Aim for this amount of nuts: one ounce two to five times per week.

A meta-analysis from 2010 examined trials that involved giving either nuts or no nuts to people who ate diets with equal amounts of saturated fats. It was the first time that we clearly saw a benefit from eating nuts. The difference was noted as a drop in total cholesterol (5 percent) and a reduction in LDL cholesterol (7 percent).[42] The study also noted that the response was dose-related; in other words, the more nuts, the more significant the impact (1.3 ounces versus 2.4 to 2.6 ounces). Importantly, the study also showed that the greatest impact was seen in people who replaced their saturated fats with nuts rather than using nuts to replace olive oil or carbohydrates. So, this shows us that if we continue to eat a Western diet full of saturated fats, exchanging those fats for nuts is of benefit. In people who already have a low saturated fat diet, the impact is less.

What is the best nut? Walnuts are known to be high in fiber and rich in antioxidants, and are a plant-based source of alpha-linolenic acid, an omega-3 fatty acid. There are studies on walnuts that show improvement in the dilation of blood vessels when given to men in exchange for one-third of their monounsaturated fats.[43]

Peanuts, which are actually legumes, are rich in monounsaturated fat, magnesium, and folate. Studies show that dietary fiber, arginine (an amino acid), and magnesium increased in a group of people eating peanuts, which may improve cardiovascular outcomes.[44]

Cashews are abundant in magnesium. Brazil nuts contain selenium, which may help to protect against prostate cancer, and deficiencies in selenium can cause weakening of the heart. Almonds are rich in fiber, vitamin E, and monounsaturated fats. They also have been shown to decrease LDL by small numbers and improve other cardiovascular parameters.[45]

There also is data to show that pecans, hazelnuts, macadamia nuts, and pistachios all have lipid-lowering abilities. But which one should you eat? Truthfully, we have read all the trials. There is data on many of the nuts. If we had to choose one nut that was better than the rest, we would probably pick the walnut. But other than that, we also think that all nuts have some benefit. (See Consider 6.) So the bottom line is that nuts are a good addition to our diets. They are best when they are used instead of oils, dairy, and meats. They are a great addition to a whole-food, plant-based diet. We should eat about a handful three to five times per week, and that is likely adequate. Overall, nuts are great but they are very calorie dense, and it is easy to overeat them. (Dr. A, for instance, has a cashew problem!) It is best to keep the amount of nuts you eat per day to a small handful. If you put out a daily portion of nuts in a container and make that the allotted amount, the tendency to overeat them is greatly reduced.

CONSIDER 6

✓ What is the best nut? Probably the walnut, but all nuts have some benefits.

What About Seeds?

Seeds are plant foods that are rich in protein. Again, few studies have been done on seeds, so unfortunately, we have little data at this point. Chia seeds and flaxseeds are probably the best seeds you can eat. Chia seeds date back to 3500 BC during the time of the Aztecs, who ate them regularly, and are abundant in fiber, calcium, and manganese. They also are the seed with the most alpha-linolenic acid (ALA), which you may recall has benefits for the heart, perhaps as a precursor for omega-3 fatty acids. In the Lyon Heart Study that looked at the Mediterranean diet, it was shown that the diet was rich in ALA, which significantly lowered heart disease risk.[46,47] Importantly, in that study, the benefits from the ALA were found apart from the benefits from fish (a marine source of omega-3 fatty acids), suggesting that the benefits from the ALA were additive.

How to eat chia seeds? Small studies show that grinding chia seeds boosts the levels of omega-3 fatty acids in the blood. They also have been associated with higher energy and a feeling of fullness. Eating a teaspoon, ground, a few times per week is probably adequate. (See Consider 7.) Similar to chia seeds, flaxseeds have also been eaten for centuries. They bring many benefits. They are also rich in alpha-linolenic acid and contain lignans, which are plant estrogens that may play a role in reducing the risk of breast cancer, at least in laboratory animals. Lignans appear to be anti-inflammatory, as well, and have been shown in small studies to lower cholesterol levels. Flaxseeds keep best when whole, but they should be ground before eating in order to get their maximum potency. One teaspoon of ground seeds a couple of times per week is likely adequate.

CONSIDER 7

✓ How to eat chia seeds? Grind your seeds to increase the absorption of omega-3 fatty acids in the blood. Have 1 teaspoon of ground chia seeds a few times per week.

Before we continue, we want to caution readers on portion sizes and how often we should eat nuts and seeds. We do not feel a person should be eating one teaspoon of chia seeds, walnuts, or flaxseed every day. All foods should be varied. We are giving general parameters. Do not eat all of these things every day because you don't need that much, and people are often frustrated with weight gain. *Vary it up!*

What about other seeds? Pumpkin seeds are high in protein and fiber. They also are rich in L-tryptophan, which can help with moods and depression. They are also rich in most B-complex vitamins (not B_{12}, however). Pomegranate seeds are also important seeds. Pomegranate has been shown in studies to decrease plaque formation in blood vessels (thus reducing heart disease). Sesame seeds are also high in fiber and calcium and are full of lignans, similar to flaxseeds. Sunflower seeds are rich in vitamin E and plant sterols, which appear to lower cholesterol. Cumin seeds, which have been used for centuries, have antiseptic properties. (See Consider 8.)

☑ People often don't think about adding seeds to their diets. Remember them when making a salad to bulk up the salad. Add to breads, cereals, and cold soups. They can be added to smoothies too!

People often want to know how much to take and how often. At the end of the day, there is no cocktail recipe. These nuts and seeds should be part of a whole-grain, plant-based diet. They should be remembered for their calcium, B vitamins, and fiber. They should be remembered as rich in alpha-linolenic acid and lignans.

A Brief Note on Children

hile caution needs to be used with adults, we believe there is more room for flexibility with children. While we prefer they don't eat oils and animal products, they do need more caloric density than their adult counterparts. So, don't hold back on nuts, seeds, and avocado for your children; it is probably okay for them to have a little oil if that is easier for food preparation. Just use the oil in moderation for children, and make up the caloric density with nuts and seeds.

People often ask Dr. A if she raises her children exclusively on a whole-grain, plant-based diet. Dr A: "The answer is that at home I cook exclusively plant-based. I feed them lots of lentils, beans, and greens. Initially, I would tell them they had to eat the food that I prepared because it was healthy. Now, they love the food. It takes trying 10 times to love something. Now my kids ask for spinach, hummus, and lentils. But if the kids go to a birthday party and eat macaroni and cheese or chicken, or we go out to dinner, I don't stop them. I am not running a dictatorship and forcing them to eat a diet that they will later rebel against. Kids need to figure it out themselves. We offer them a healthy lifestyle at home, and I hope that, with time, they will realize the difference in how they feel when they eat the foods that are good for them. Truthfully, with a few exceptions, my kids love to eat plant-based!"

A healthy diet is not about any one food. It is not about eating three grams of fish oil or flaxseeds. It is not only about kale or limiting yourself to eating just walnuts or vegetables. It is also not about eating high-fat, processed foods and then adding nuts or kale and expect to make it all better. It is about the whole thing. When people try to tease out what is great about the Mediterranean diet, a plant-based diet, or any diet for that matter, they often are looking for that one magic food that is going to heal them. We have to put work into this lifestyle and learn how to complement foods, so we get a balanced diet. Magic foods don't exist. There is no one ingredient that makes our health better. It is the whole thing—a balance. Once we understand that, then true healing can begin.

YOUR PRESCRIPTION

FINDING YOUR GOOD FOOD BALANCE

1. Try to decrease oil intake in general. No oil is really good for you. Try to be creative by using water or orange juice to sauté.

2. If you want to add oil for taste, the best oil is probably flaxseed oil. However, you cannot heat flaxseed oil because it makes the good fats unhealthy. It's best to use flaxseeds in baking or add them to morning cereal, shakes, or oatmeal. Consider eating them in a salad.

3. Canola and olive oils are probably the best oils to cook with. But remember, there are no wonder oils.

4. If you feel as if you need more substance, eat nuts, seeds, and avocado. They are calorie-dense and will make you feel full, but too many will cause weight gain.

5. There is no magic food. There is no food you can eat that will balance out the bad foods you're eating. Eat balanced. Be creative and learn how to make fabulous food that is tasty and great for you.

CHAPTER

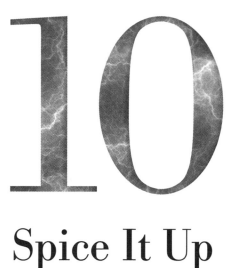

Spice It Up

WITH THE SPICES (AND HERBS) OF LIFE

The flavorful and ancient anti-inflammatory medicine cabinet in our kitchens

S pices are an essential part of any diet. They are very potent in decreasing inflammation and have many medicinal properties. Spices have been an important part of life for millennia, long praised for their flavors, aromas, and medicinal properties. There are Egyptian documents tracing the use of spices as early as 2000 to 1500 BCE showing how the role of spices as medicine was appreciated. These documents note the benefits of anise, mustard, saffron, and cinnamon. Egyptians used cinnamon for mummification. Cinnamon was put in vials and placed in pharaohs' coffins to accompany them to the afterlife. Notably, cinnamon is not endemic to ancient Egypt, suggesting spice trading occurred that long ago.

Notes written in 950 BCE mention an incense route followed by traders carrying spices from Asia to Europe. Spices were coveted and traded for large sums of gold and silver. When Alexander the Great conquered Egypt in 80 BCE, he established Alexandria in Egypt as a port for spice trade. Romans and Greeks viewed spices as markers of wealth and luxury; they would heap them on banquet tables and use them in making spice-scented perfumes. They also valued the medicinal properties of spices. During the eighth to fifteenth centuries, spice trade was an important form of commerce dominated by the republic of Venice. Spices were moved from Asia to Europe with the help of Arab middlemen.[1]

In the fifteenth century, Spain and Portugal attempted to thwart the Venetian monopoly and sent Christopher Columbus to find India via a western route. It was on that trip that he discovered America. Over the following centuries, the Dutch, Spanish, French, and British colonized all the countries that could provide an abundance of spices. By the end of the seventeenth century, the Dutch East India Company was the richest corporation in the world, showing how much spices were valued.

Why are spices so valued? Because of their potential role in health. Spices are concentrated forms of the most potent parts of the plants they come from. Spices are full of phytonutrients. Recall, phytonutrients are involved in cell signaling and communication, the information pathway in the body. We have established that phytonutrients are found in fruits and vegetables. However, some phytonutrients can be found only in spices. When phytonutrients are involved in cell signaling, they have the potential to turn inflammatory cascades on and off. In that way, spices can be beneficial in reducing inflammation and oxidative stresses.

So what do spices contain that can be found nowhere else? Curcumin, a vital anti-inflammatory with anticancer benefits, can only be found in turmeric. Thymoquinone is a potent immune booster and only exists in black cumin. Piperine has neuroprotective effects (protects the brain cells) and is unique to black pepper. Eugenol, found only in cloves, is a powerful painkiller. Rosmarinic acid is a potent antioxidant, and the only source is rosemary. Capsaicin is a great medication for arthritis, and its only source is chili peppers. The list goes on and on.

The data on the benefits of spices is not optimal. Small animal studies are all we have to go on. But we think the potential benefits based on those studies is encouraging. Let's talk about a few of our favorites. (See figure 1 on the next page.)

FIGURE 1	Certain Phytonutrients can only be found in spices

SPICES	ACTIVE INGREDIENTS	ACTION
Black Cumin	Thymoquinone	Immune Booster
Turmeric	Curcumin	Anti-Inflammatory
Black Pepper	Piperine	Protects Brain Cells
Cloves	Eugenol	Pain Killer
Rosemary	Rosmarinic Acid	Anti-Oxidant
Chili	Capsaicin	Pain Reliever

Turmeric—Our Gold

F or centuries, the people of India have been studied because until recently they suffered very little chronic illness. Yes, diseases of poverty and poor medical attention are rampant, but chronic illness was not—at least it wasn't until the modern era. This is likely because of something called the thrift theory: For centuries, Indian people lived in villages and walked as their form of transportation. They subsisted on diets consisting primarily of rice, vegetables, nuts, seeds, and spices. Turmeric is one of the spices that is used widely in that country, and it has many potential benefits.

Turmeric's vital ingredient is curcumin, and it appears to have anti-inflammatory properties. In small studies, turmeric has been shown to decrease inflammation in joints and reduce symptoms of arthritis. In a recent study, one group of participants took 2,000 milligrams of turmeric compared to participants who took 800 milligrams of ibuprofen. Researchers found that turmeric provided at least as much relief from peoples' symptoms as ibuprofen and without the side effects that come from taking anti-inflammatory medications.[2] How cool is that! (See Consider 1.)

Turmeric may also be a powerful antioxidant. It has been shown in animal studies to lower risk of cancers, such as breast, colon, prostate, and even skin cancers, when ingested regularly. The incidence of cancer in India is much lower than in the West.[3]

Turmeric may also play a role in treating Alzheimer's disease, due to the spice's anti-inflammatory effects. Alzheimer's disease affects 5 to 6 percent of the population older than 60 years of age worldwide and 10 percent of the American population over 65 years.[4] The number in the US is expected to quadruple by the year 2050. Our brains contain cells called neurons that are responsible for making connections so that our thoughts can manifest in actions. But in people with Alzheimer's disease, plaque forms between these cells, reducing the ability of these neurons to communicate. These communications are the key to cognition, memory, and judgment, and without these functions we see the impairments evident in Alzheimer's patients. Triggers for Alzheimer's disease are likely related to inflammation and oxidative stress.

Because of curcumin's known anti-inflammatory and antioxidant effects, animal studies have been conducted on its effects on Alzheimer's disease. In experiments using mice, there was a 40 percent reduction in plaque in mice treated with curcumin, which is an unbelievable reduction.[5] Notably, small doses over a long period of time were more effective than large doses in a short period of time, suggesting the benefit is long term and the spice needs to be eaten over the long term as well. Consider, then, the impact of eating turmeric over a lifetime.

Curcumin is also an important antiviral and antiseptic. For centuries, people have applied turmeric paste to cuts to prevent bacterial infections. It might even have cardiovascular benefits; in studies on mice, fewer fatty deposits were found in those eating turmeric. Researchers also found notably less LDL and less overall inflammation.[6] Similarly, a recent article compared rabbits that ate a high-cholesterol meal and turmeric with those that ate a high-cholesterol meal without the spice. The rabbits that ate the added turmeric had less atherosclerotic plaque than their counterparts. The authors concluded that the effects of turmeric were multifaceted and included lowering both cholesterol and inflammatory markers.[7]

We feel that turmeric is like gold. We use it regularly in our cooking, and Dr A's husband makes her morning tea with turmeric in it every day.

Rosemary—the Cancer Fighter

Herbs, too, can be important health boosters, and one we love is rosemary. Rosemary has three essential components: rosmarinic acid, carnosic acid, and carnosol. These elements are potent antioxidants. When we cook food on a grill at high temperatures and the food burns, it releases toxic chemicals called heterocyclic amines (HCAs). (See page 56.) Traces of HCAs are found in breast, prostate, and colon cancers. When we place rosemary on the grill with our food, studies show that the amount of HCAs decreases. In a recent study, when rosemary extract was added to beef, HCA production was inhibited by 85 to 91 percent![8] Similarly, mice that were injected with carcinogens (cancer-causing chemicals) and also received carnosol (a component of rosemary) developed 61 percent fewer tumors. (See Consider 2.)

CONSIDER 2

✔ Bring sprigs of rosemary to your next barbecue. Throw them onto the grill along with your other foods. They add great flavor and help decrease cancer risk.

Rosemary has been around for centuries. There are references to it in the Bible. Early Greeks and Romans used it as a funeral decoration. Even simply smelling rosemary has been found to decrease cortisol (a stress hormone). Rosemary is an important herb for its anticancer benefits, and it's one we try to use regularly in our diets.

Cinnamon—the Sweet Non-Sugar That Helps Lower Sugar in Your Blood

As we have discussed, because there is less emphasis on exercise, sleep, and good diet, many chronic illnesses have become epidemic in modern society. Diabetes and cardiovascular disease are rampant. Cinnamon is an important spice in treating diabetes; it's a good antioxidant and important in enhancing insulin sensitivity. Recall that in diabetes, the body does not respond to the insulin that is present, so sugar is not converted to fat—which is the main purpose of insulin. Sugar then circulates in the blood and increases risk for forming plaque in the heart. We have studies that show the benefits of adding cinnamon to foods to decrease blood sugars. When diabetic patients were given one gram, three grams, or six grams of cinnamon, all groups showed improvement in blood sugar, triglycerides, LDL, and total cholesterol compared to a control group. Interestingly, there was no dose-dependent relationship, meaning it didn't matter which dose people took because they all experienced a significant, similar drop in sugar and cholesterol levels within about 40 days.[9]

People with diabetes, however, aren't the only ones who are rewarded for eating cinnamon. In one study, animals given high-fat or high-sugar diets and cinnamon were less likely to develop insulin resistance (an indicator of prediabetes) than those not given the cinnamon.[10] This suggests that the benefits of cinnamon extend beyond treating diabetes and can be useful in decreasing one's risk of developing diabetes as well.

Cinnamon is also an antifungal agent.[11] It has antibacterial properties as well, with studies showing it is effective in combating molds, stomach bugs, and common pneumonias.[12] Cinnamon is effective in killing oral bacteria—which is why we see cinnamon in chewing gum.[13] It also improves circulation and is a key ingredient in Tiger Balm, an herbal cream used to ease sore joints. Another important benefit is its effect as an antioxidant. Small studies suggest that cinnamon oils can help remove free radicals, which are responsible for attacking our cells and creating cancers.[14] (See Consider 3.)

CONSIDER 3

 Add cinnamon to your baked foods instead of sugar to sweeten them. It can potentially lower your blood sugar level.

Garlic—the Stinking Rose

arlic, the "stinking rose," is actually a vegetable, but people often think of it as an herb. Historically, documents have been retrieved from 3,500 years ago that claim garlic can be effective in treating heart disease.[15] Why is garlic so great? It's nutrient-rich; it's 65 percent water and the remainder is carbohydrates, protein, fiber, and free amino acids. Garlic is loaded with potassium, phosphorus, zinc, and selenium. It's known for its abundance of saponins, which are responsible for fighting against bacteria that might attack the plant. Like plants, which use saponins to fight off bacteria, we believe humans can harness saponins and benefit from their antibacterial effects. Saponins are also believed to be effective anticancer treatments. (See Consider 4.)

CONSIDER 4

✓ Add garlic to all your foods to help with heart disease. If you are coming down with a stomach bug, think about taking some garlic.

Phenols are antioxidants found in fruits, vegetables, and spices. Garlic is rich in phenols, so it is a potent antioxidant. Many studies have been done on garlic's lipid-lowering abilities. About half of the studies were negative, but in the half that showed a benefit, the payoff was seen in people with the higher cholesterol levels. In those cases, LDL cholesterol and triglycerides dropped by about 10 percent when participants ate garlic.[16] Other studies showed that in both normal subjects and those with high cholesterol, garlic had some effect in reducing platelet aggregation. Recall, platelet aggregation can create plaque formation. Further studies show that garlic also improves the elasticity of our blood vessels. Elasticity is a good thing because it allows blood vessels to change based on blood flow requirements.[17]

What kind of garlic is best? The answer is unclear. In the trials, many formulations were used. Some trials showed that aged garlic was superior, but that isn't conclusive. Our bottom line is eat garlic frequently because its benefits are short-acting. Don't worry so much about which garlic is better—just eat it. Fresh is always best.

Our Spice Cabinet

T here are so many delicious and aromatic spices with potential health benefits. We wanted to highlight some of our favorites, but on a daily basis, we try to get an abundance of spices into our diets. We regularly use cumin, coriander powder, pomegranate powder, ajowan (popular in Indian dishes), mango powder, and black pepper. As you start your meal preparations, open your spice cupboard and consider which spices you could add to the recipe.

YOUR PRESCRIPTION

FINDING THE SPICE OF YOUR LIFE

1. Try to be creative by adding a little spice into all of your meals. Try different combinations and experience the flavors.

2. Eat turmeric at least a few times each week. Add black pepper to help its absorption. Turmeric is bitter, so start by adding it gradually to stews, beans, and soups until you become more comfortable with it. Now, we add it to our drinking water for flavor. Add ¼–½ teaspoon turmeric and ⅛ teaspoon ground black pepper to 20 ounces of water. Add a splash of lemon.

3. Adding spices is a great way to get flavor without adding salt. If you have high blood pressure or have been told to restrict your salt intake, think about using cumin, garlic, and black pepper to flavor your foods.

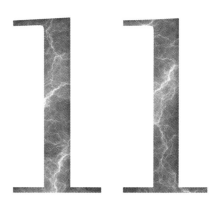

Water

THE ESSENCE OF LIFE

Water, an integral part of our existence

Our bodies are 60 percent water. It is an essential component of the body's fluids, including blood, synovial fluid (fluid around the joints), saliva, digestive juices, lymph fluids, urine, sweat, and tears. Water is also a part of every internal organ and system in the body. Those organs and systems need adequate water to operate effectively. The nervous system relies on fluids for communication. Our digestive, lymph, and reproductive systems all rely on water for proper functioning. Every cell in our bodies needs water because water is the vehicle that distributes the electrolytes necessary for creating energy, transfers nutrients into cells, and removes debris from the cells. Every bodily function requires water at some level.

Water is also critical for maintaining proper body temperature. When we feel hot, we sweat out water through our skin, and when it evaporates, the body is able to cool itself. Sweating is also a form of detoxification. Water helps the stomach, eyes, mouth, and throat stay moist by keeping the mucosal lining hydrated. (See figure 1 on the next page.)

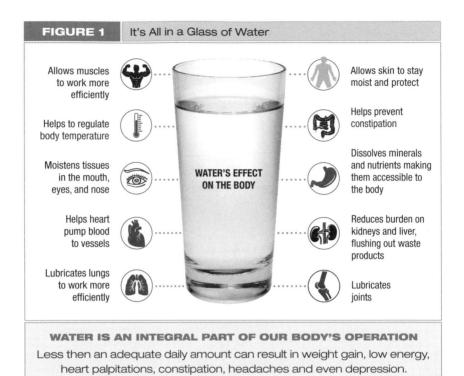

FIGURE 1   It's All in a Glass of Water

Allows muscles to work more efficiently

Helps to regulate body temperature

Moistens tissues in the mouth, eyes, and nose

Helps heart pump blood to vessels

Lubricates lungs to work more efficiently

WATER'S EFFECT ON THE BODY

Allows skin to stay moist and protect

Helps prevent constipation

Dissolves minerals and nutrients making them accessible to the body

Reduces burden on kidneys and liver, flushing out waste products

Lubricates joints

WATER IS AN INTEGRAL PART OF OUR BODY'S OPERATION

Less then an adequate daily amount can result in weight gain, low energy, heart palpitations, constipation, headaches and even depression.

Every day, our bodies lose water through respiration (think of your foggy breath on a cold winter day), urination, sweating, and fecal material, resulting in approximately 2.4 liters (just over 80 ounces) of water lost each and every day. Losses are then balanced by what we take in. We obtain our fluids from what we drink and the liquid in our food. Drinking water is the easiest way to hydrate our bodies. Eating water-rich fruits and vegetables is also a great way to keep hydrated.

When the brain detects that we lack water, it activates our thirst mechanism. If we don't quench our thirst, not only does our urine become dark in color, but our stools also become hard, and we become constipated. Without fluids, some people feel faint and lightheaded. Others get headaches. With persistent dehydration, the kidneys start failing. People can develop palpitations (heart flutters), which resolve with fluid intake. We use hydration to maintain blood pressure.

A dehydrated body is a stressed body, and stress is a major source of disease. A healthy body can live for several weeks without food, but it cannot survive more than several days without water. Severe dehydration for an extended time can kill you. Many people do not understand that coffee, sodas, juices, and many energy drinks have a dehydrating effect on the body and do not replenish our bodies. Sodas, tea, coffee, and juices are also not good options for hydration because they have so many other ingredients. The sugars in juice and caffeine in tea cause us to urinate without actually hydrating us. Most people simply do not consume enough water or foods with a high water content.

Dehydration also can contribute to weight gain and obesity. People often confuse dehydration with hunger. Often, when we feel our stomachs rumbling, we reach for food when, in fact, we are simply thirsty and need to drink some water. People also choose to consume high-caloric drinks, such as sodas, fruit juices, and energy drinks, instead of water, adding to weight gain. Our metabolisms will actually slow down when we are dehydrated, thus we will burn fewer calories, again raising the potential for weight gain.[1] (See Consider 1.)

CONSIDER 1

☑ When you're hungry, try drinking a glass of water before you start eating something.

☑ People can confuse dehydration with hunger; drinking a glass of water can dissipate our desire to eat.

Many of our clients are successful in changing their food choices, and they start losing unwanted weight. Drinking more water, especially before a meal, helps increase weight loss. (See Consider 2.)

CONSIDER 2

Coffee, sodas, juices, and energy drinks have a dehydrating effect on the body.

1. What percent of your daily liquid intake is actually water versus other beverages?

2. Try tracking the number of glasses of water you drink in one day. Note: a glass holds almost two cups of water. *Some experts believe you should drink eight cups (64 ounces) of water per day.*

People often ask about the optimal amount to drink, but no one really knows the answer. Some experts say we should drink eight cups of water per day. We don't really know if that is the best quantity, and many believe that even more would be beneficial. People complain, though, that they have to go to the bathroom too often when they drink enough water—but urinating frequently is a good thing. Remember, your kidneys are excreting toxins in your urine, so it is good to go to the bathroom more often. Just keep an eye on the color of the urine and gauge if you are drinking enough.

So our recommendation is to drink water often and in larger quantities. Avoid sodas and juices, which are empty calories and don't hydrate you. If you enjoy tea and coffee, understand that you're not hydrating, and drink water along with your caffeinated drinks. Your goal should be to urinate every two hours. There is no recommended amount of water to drink. Listen to your body. Listen to your thirst. Get yourself a 20-ounce bottle, fill it full of water, and drink the entire bottle three to four times a day. You will be refreshed.

YOUR PRESCRIPTION

1. Drink water often and in fairly large amounts each day.

2. There is no substitute for water.

3. Think about when you urinated last. Has it been a while? You should try to urinate once every couple of hours. Look at your urine. If it is dark, you need to go back and drink more water.

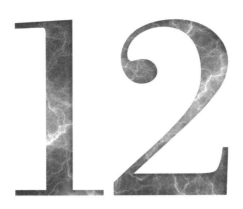

Sleep On It

Rejuvenate and detoxify by catching some Z's

Dr. R: When my third child was just five weeks old, I received a frantic phone call from my older son's second grade teacher. The teacher had noticed an issue with my son over the past three weeks, and she was concerned. He had become easily distracted, was not following directions, and was not completing classwork assignments, which was a big departure from the past. She felt he was showing signs of ADHD and recommended that I seek medical attention for him.

The following week, my son picked up a soccer ball in the middle of a game when he was not playing the goalie position. This concerned his coach, who had worked with him for three years. My husband and I were starting to worry about these new symptoms of distraction, and, feeling very frustrated, my husband asked, "What is wrong with you?" Our son replied with equal frustration in his voice, "It's not like I have slept since the baby was born!" It was then I realized my son was suffering from poor sleep because of the daily disruptions from the baby. He hadn't had a good night's sleep in weeks. We moved my son to another bedroom so he couldn't hear the baby crying at night, and the very next day, he woke up refreshed and feeling like himself again. Within days, his concentration and strange behavior had resolved.

Sleep—It's Not Just About Being Tired

S leep disorders affect 50 to 70 million Americans. Unfortunately, inadequate sleep is common in our society. The most obvious symptom is daytime fatigue; over time it can cause a depressed mood, irritability, and poor concentration. Lack of sleep can also lead to difficulty with weight loss and metabolic issues, such as diabetes and hypertension. In addition, it also has a significant impact on a person's safety. Those who sleep less than eight hours are two to four times more likely to be involved in a car crash than those who sleep more.[1] The National Sleep Foundation recommends that adults ages 18 to 64 get between seven and nine hours of restorative sleep in order to maintain health.[2]

As early as the eighteenth century, it was understood that there was a cyclical nature to a day that was 24 hours long and corresponded to the Earth's rotation. This rotation also connects to the biological clock in our cells, leading to a circadian rhythm. Circadian rhythms are the biological, physical, and behavioral changes that occur with a 24-hour sleep/wake cycle. The circadian rhythm is set to environmental cues, such as the rising and setting of the sun. Researchers have more recently discovered that hormones such as cortisol (that stress hormone again) also are affected by that same cycle. Recall, cortisol is our wake-up hormone; it takes cues from external sources, such as sunlight, and is at its peak in the early morning.

During daylight hours, we have higher levels of cortisol. These levels subside as the day progresses, and as cortisol wanes, levels of adenosine and melatonin increase. Adenosine is a chemical that increases during the day and promotes sleepiness as the day goes on. As evening approaches and the light disappears, melatonin also increases and prepares our body for sleep. Melatonin is often considered our sleep hormone because it works to synchronize our biological clocks. Melatonin is released when it gets dark, and the amount in our system peaks at around 2:00 a.m. to 4:00 a.m. On the other hand, when we are asleep, our bodies break down adenosine, and it drops to a low level in the morning. Low levels of adenosine promote wakefulness. Since we know that melatonin promotes sleeping, it makes sense that people take melatonin supplements to regulate their sleep.

With a sleep deficit, cortisol breaks down more slowly. Therefore, when we don't sleep, these stress hormones remain at a higher level.

Recall that higher levels of stress hormones (chronic distress) over time can lead to inflammation. More on this later.

How Much Sleep Do We Need?

leep requirements change as we age.[3] Newborns sleep most of the time—8 to 16 hours per day. As they reach the toddler stage, children sleep 11 to 13 hours and need frequent naps. According to the National Sleep Foundation, children require from 10 to 13 hours in their younger years (ages three to five), and by the time they become preteens they need 9 to 11 hours.

When children become teenagers, they still require 8 to 10 hours of sleep per night. How many of our high school students actually sleep that much, given their late nights and early wake-up alarms? Adults and seniors require 7 to 9 hours of sleep per day. Do you get enough sleep? Does it matter if you don't? (See Consider 1 below and figure 1 on the next page.)

CONSIDER 1

☑ Do you get enough sleep?

☑ How many hours would you sleep if the alarm did not wake you up?

☑ Do you feel rested when you wake up?

Stages of Sleep

n a normal cycle, we go through several stages of sleep—usually at least one stage of REM (rapid eye movement) and four stages of non-REM sleep. REM sleep is a time of low muscle tone and rapid eye movements. This cycle lasts about 90 minutes and recurs frequently through the night. The REM sleep cycle increases in length as sleep continues through the night. REM sleep is the time when people dream the most vividly. About 50 percent of a baby's sleeping hours are REM, but for adults REM time shrinks to about 20 percent. The full benefit of these individual stages is not entirely clear, but we do know that all stages are necessary. Restorative sleep requires four to five cycles of all stages of non-REM and REM sleep. If we don't get that sleep, we call that *sleep debt*, which can be associated with multiple health issues that we will discuss later.

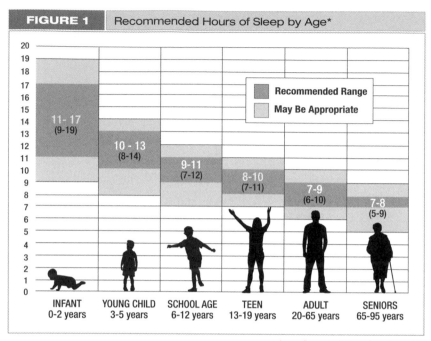

FIGURE 1 Recommended Hours of Sleep by Age*

Recommended Range
May Be Appropriate

INFANT 0-2 years: 11-17 (9-19)
YOUNG CHILD 3-5 years: 10-13 (8-14)
SCHOOL AGE 6-12 years: 9-11 (7-12)
TEEN 13-19 years: 8-10 (7-11)
ADULT 20-65 years: 7-9 (6-10)
SENIORS 65-95 years: 7-8 (5-9)

*according to the National Sleep Foundation

Seniors in general struggle with sleep and often suffer from sleep debt. Along with the physical changes that occur as we get older, changes to our sleep patterns are a part of the normal aging process. As people age, they tend to have a harder time falling asleep and more trouble staying asleep than when they were younger. However, it is a common misconception that as we age, we need less sleep. In fact, research demonstrates that our sleep needs remain constant throughout adulthood. So, what's keeping seniors awake? Often, it is a mechanical problem, such as a need to urinate, medication side effects, or a complication of a physical or psychiatric illness. Interestingly, though, older people spend more time in the lighter stages of sleep than in deep sleep.

Many older adults also report being less satisfied with sleep and more tired during the day. Studies on the sleep habits of older Americans show an increase in the time it takes to fall asleep (sleep latency), an overall decline in REM sleep, and an increase in sleep fragmentation (waking up during the night) with age. Naps during the day may work to eliminate sleepiness, but they cannot reverse all of the detrimental effects of disruptive sleep.

Many modern environmental factors provoke sleep debt. First, some of us have to work night shifts several times a week. Shift work or any other forced change in our clocks, such as being caregivers at night, can disrupt our circadian rhythms. We also travel, often for work, at all hours of the day to places in different time zones. We are then forced to operate on a different time clock without any opportunity to restore our systems.

Many of us stay up late to finish chores or to just get some alone time before we turn in. We have trouble going to bed at 10:00 p.m. because we have things we want to do. But in order to get eight hours of sleep before the alarm wakes us at 6:00 a.m, our sleep rituals have to start in a timely manner the night before. Most of us check emails and social media late into the night. Then there are the late-night television shows and shows previously taped. Even after we're asleep, our tablets and phones buzz all night and interrupt our rest. Does this sound familiar? To most of us, it does. All of these activities impact our natural circadian rhythm. The unnatural light lowers our melatonin levels. (See Consider 2.)

CONSIDER 2

☑ How late do you check your email?

☑ What is the last thing you do before you sleep?

☑ Is your mind racing because you just watched the news or due to an email that you just read?

Medical illnesses can also create sleep debt. Neurodegenerative conditions such as dementia, Parkinson's disease, pain, anxiety, and depression can cause sleep interruption. Benign prostate hypertrophy (BPH), a benign condition that causes the prostate gland to enlarge in men and as a result causes frequent urination, or pelvic floor weakening in women (after multiple children) also deprive us of sleep. Menopause, too, is often associated with sleep disruption. Sleep apnea, which causes a person to stop breathing at night for short periods, causes disrupted sleep as the body wakes up to breathe. Certain medications, such as antidepressants, also can act like stimulants, which increase nighttime arousal. Stimulants, such as caffeine, tea, chocolate, and sodas, can keep our systems activated for up to eight hours and prevent us from calming down enough to sleep. Nicotine from cigarettes also can keep us activated late into the night. (See Consider 3.)

(See Consider 3.)

CONSIDER 3

☑ Do you have trouble sleeping at night?

☑ Do you take in any stimulants, such as tea, coffee, or chocolate, in the afternoon?

Sleep and Our Stress Hormones— The Link Between Stress and Cortisol

E arlier we mentioned that cortisol levels should be highest in the morning and decrease throughout the day. During the evening, we have higher levels of adenosine and melatonin, which help us sleep. Sleep deprivation has a major impact on stress hormone regulation through two pathways: activity at the brain level and through the autonomic nervous system (the nervous system in charge of our stress response).

The pituitary gland is considered the master endocrine gland and controls secretion of several hormones. During normal sleep patterns, growth hormone is released, emphasizing the need for better sleep in order to grow. Normally, while we sleep, cortisol production is decreased. When sleep deprivation occurs, however, it causes a stress response, and the sympathetic nervous system (fight or flight) is activated.[3] Our adrenaline increases, and we are ready to get moving. With chronic sleep deprivation, our hormone balance is disrupted. One study illustrates this concept. It looked at eleven men who slept four to six hours per night and noted that those with this sleep debt had higher evening cortisol levels and higher activation of the sympathetic nervous system than their counterparts who slept more.[3]

Sleep debt, then, is a distress to our bodies (see pages 17–21) similar to chronic stress. We see increases in our inflammatory markers with sleep debt as well (tumor necrosis factor and Interleukin 6).[5] These markers are part of the immune system defense, and they respond to enemies such as viral infections and tumors. They help the body fight foreign cells by creating symptoms, such as a fever, and recruit-

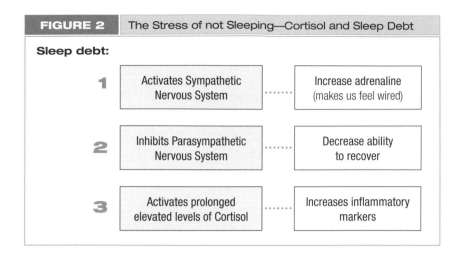

FIGURE 2   The Stress of not Sleeping—Cortisol and Sleep Debt

Sleep debt:

1 Activates Sympathetic Nervous System · · · · · · · · Increase adrenaline (makes us feel wired)

2 Inhibits Parasympathetic Nervous System · · · · · · · · Decrease ability to recover

3 Activates prolonged elevated levels of Cortisol · · · · · · · · Increases inflammatory markers

ing other fighter cells into the areas where there is inflammation—*a good thing*. However, in the presence of chronic inflammation from persistent sleep loss, these markers can be persistently elevated and cause symptoms of fatigue and sluggishness—*a bad thing*. (See figure 2 and Consider 4.)

CONSIDER 4

Consider how much faster you recover from a cold or virus when you give yourself enough time to sleep.

Sleep as an Antioxidant

Another very important aspect of sleep is its antioxidant potential. In order for the body to work, it needs oxygen. However, the use of oxygen in cellular reactions can generate free radicals, which make our cells unstable and cause damage to our DNA. Consequently, this can lead to chronic illness, including creating a focal point for cancer-causing cells. Multiple triggers for this free radical formation have been discussed in previous chapters. Antioxidants are needed to protect our cells against damage from this oxidative stress. Sleep deprivation adversely affects the immune system, creates even higher oxidative stress, and in turn contributes to even more metabolic imbalances.[6,7] In contrast, sleep is restorative and serves as an antioxidant.

Glutathione, produced by the liver, is one of the strongest antioxidants in our bodies. We've learned that as little as five days of sleep deprivation can impair the production of glutathione by 30 percent.[8] Studies also show that a glutathione depletion of 20 to 30 percent can impair cellular defense systems and lead to abnormal cell-to-cell communication, and cause adverse effects to protein breakdown and cell injury.[9] In an animal study, sleep deprivation accelerated glutathione depletion, which showed an increase in cell damage in heart tissue. However, sleep recovery showed restoration of glutathione and antioxidant activity in both liver and heart.[10]

It has been shown that the immune system works best if there are balanced levels of glutathione. This has been studied most extensively in individuals with HIV (human immunodeficiency virus) infection where there is a severe immune system dysfunction as a result of the virus attacking immune T lymphocyte cells. In those studies, people who took glutathione-like compounds had significant increases in their immunological functions.[11] More research is needed, but this may be another reason we see immune dysfunction (such as increased colds) with sleep deprivation. (See Consider 5.)

CONSIDER 5

✓ Glutathione is an effective antioxidant and increases with more sleep.

Sleep Debt and Performance

Impaired performance can affect your personal safety, as well as efficiency at work or play. As we sleep less and become more sleep deprived, our diminished alertness translates into more workplace errors and higher numbers of auto accidents in which drivers fall asleep at the wheel.[12]

Studies have looked at daytime alertness in the workplace as well. David Dinges, PhD, head of the Sleep and Chronology Laboratory at the University of Pennsylvania, divided dozens of people into three groups for a two-week period: those who slept for four hours, six hours, and eight hours. He did psychomotor testing, which involved subjects performing simple tasks, such as pressing the space bar of a computer when they noted a certain symbol on the computer. He found that those people who slept eight hours had no difficulty with their psychomotor testing, whereas both the four-hour and six-hour sleep groups showed significant declines in their psychomotor performance over the two-week period.[13]

At the halfway point of the study, 25 percent of the six-hour group was falling asleep at the computer. They had trouble with basic math questions and cognitive skills. By the end of the study, performance reduced significantly. A *New York Times* article about the study read, "Six-hour sleepers were as impaired as those who, in another Dinges study, had been sleep-deprived for 24 hours straight—the cognitive equivalent of being legally drunk."[14, 15] It was noted that seven hours was not enough sleep, and cognitive testing was impaired even at that level of sleep. This sleep deprivation is what Dr. Rao believed affected her son's behavior. In fact, older studies show that if we reduce our sleep for even one night by 1.3 to 1.5 hours, our daytime alertness is decreased by 32 percent.[16] (See Consider 6.)

CONSIDER 6

✓ Even though it seems we can get more done by staying awake longer and taking that time out of our sleep, our efficiency the next day can be reduced by 32 percent. You will be better off to save the work until tomorrow and get a good night's sleep.

Sleep Debt and Disease

S tudies are mounting showing that short sleep periods, poor sleep quality, and sleep deprivation are associated with diabetes, metabolic syndrome, and obesity.[17,18,19] This can be attributed to several issues, including hormones affected by poor sleep. Insulin is one hormone that regulates glucose metabolism, the process of using sugar for energy. Sleep deprivation for as little as a week has been shown to cause changes in the body that can mimic the insulin resistance seen with type 2 diabetes.[20,21]

In one study, fasting morning glucose levels in those experiencing sleep debt (only four hours) was 15 points higher than those who had slept normally.[22] In other words, if you had slept for only four hours, your fasting sugar level in the morning was 15 points higher than someone who had slept for eight hours. Remember, fasting blood sugar is used to diagnose diabetes. Fifteen points can absolutely make a difference in whether you have the disease or you don't. As discussed on page 26, high blood sugar levels eventually lead to insulin resistance, which then can cause diabetes.

When we sleep less, it may actually shorten our lifespan! (See Consider 7.) In an observational study, men who slept for fewer than six hours had a shorter lifespan than those who slept more.[23] (This observation took into consideration hypertension and diabetes.) There also appears to be a higher incidence of other cardiovascular risk factors in sleep-deprived people, such as hypertension, obesity, diabetes, heart disease, and stroke.[24] These illnesses are likely triggered by the inflammation caused by sleep debt.

CONSIDER 7

☑ When you sleep less, you can potentially shorten your lifespan.

Appetite and Sleep

O ur appetite for high-calorie foods also increases with sleep deprivation. That trend is partly due to your body's extra demands for calories and energy, simply because you are awake longer. Several hormones associated with weight management also are affected. Ghrelin is a hormone secreted by the stomach that stimulates appetite and has been shown to increase with sleep loss. Therefore, you are hungrier when you sleep less. Leptin is the hormone that tells your body that it is full and your appetite decreases. After only two nights of sleep deprivation (only four hours), ghrelin production increased by 28 percent and leptin production decreased by 18 percent.[25] In other words, two days of sleeping four hours makes you hungrier and reduces your body's ability to know you are full.

Sleep loss also changes how we utilize energy. One study showed that sleep deprivation slowed down fat loss by 55 percent compared to a control group with similar caloric intake but no sleep deprivation.[26] This may be one reason why so many sleep-deprived people are unable to lose weight in spite of restricting their calories. (See figure 3 on the next page.)

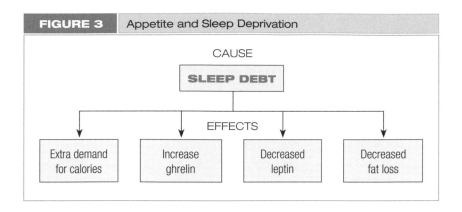

FIGURE 3 | Appetite and Sleep Deprivation

CAUSE

SLEEP DEBT

EFFECTS

| Extra demand for calories | Increase ghrelin | Decreased leptin | Decreased fat loss |

Sleep Debt and Memory

The act of learning new information requires several pathways within the hippocampus, a part of our brain critical for memory. When we make memories, we perceive smell, taste, and feelings, and these sensations are transmitted to the hippocampus and integrated. It's believed that in the hippocampus, it is decided if something perceived is worth remembering. With sleep debt, disruptions to the pathways to the hippocampus have been noted, so our memories aren't as sharp.[27]

As early as 1924, studies were done showing that retention of nonsense syllables and short stories was better with sleep than without. Many studies since have shown that sleep debt causes difficulty in memory recall. How much sleep and what stages of sleep are required for memory are unclear. More recent studies have shown that we need more non-REM sleep for memories of stories, words, and random information. You'll remember that non-REM sleep is sleep that usually occurs at the beginning of the night. Storing of emotional memories, however, appears to require more REM sleep, which occurs later in the evening.[28]

Cortisol plays a role in making memories as well. We know that during early parts of sleep, cortisol levels are at their lowest. It appears that low levels of cortisol are needed for storing memories. In studies where patients were either given hydrocortisone (a cortisol-like compound) or had high levels of cortisol due to a medical illness, notable impairments in word recall and memory were noted.[29] We also know that with sleep debt, cortisol does not break down well. Consider this cycle then: when we are stressed, we have higher cortisol levels. With higher cortisol, we have more trouble sleeping. With higher cortisol, we have less ability to retain memories.

Sleep Apnea

Sleep apnea also triggers memory loss.[30] Sleep apnea is characterized by heavy snoring and intermittent episodes of apnea, or absence of breathing. During those times of lapsed breathing, less oxygen gets to the brain and organs. The body realizes the problem and causes the person to wake up, leading to significant sleep disruption. However, the person then falls back to sleep and has more episodes of apnea. The cycle repeats over and over during the night.

Apnea is associated with hypertension and headaches, and higher rates of stroke, heart disease, abnormal heart rhythms, and heart failure. Sleep apnea directly impacts and alters endothelial function as well.[31] Recall that the endothelial cells are the cells that line our blood vessels; damage to these cells results in a cascade of inflammation and oxidative stress. The blood vessels also become impaired and can't open as well in response to more demand for blood.

CASE 1: A 50-year-old male was noted to have daytime fatigue and high CRP (marker of inflammation) elevated to 43 (normal is up to 3). He had been diagnosed with sleep apnea but was having trouble wearing his mask. He also had been working the night shift for the past five years. He shifted his night shift to day shift and started wearing his CPAP mask for his sleep apnea regularly. In six weeks, his CRP returned to normal range.

Drops in oxygen levels with sleep apnea can lead to shrinking of certain cells in our brains called mammillary bodies, which are involved with our memory and thinking. Diminished mammillary body volume in people with sleep apnea may be associated with memory loss and problems with spatial orientation. The mechanisms contributing to the loss of mammillary bodies are unclear, but may relate to a low supply of oxygen.[30]

Sleep apnea most commonly occurs in people who are overweight. It can continue to make attempted weight loss more difficult. Why? Sleep apnea can lower the metabolism, which makes weight loss challenging. Reversing sleep apnea not only improves daytime fatigue, but it also can rev up your metabolism, making it easier to lose weight. It also can reverse many of the cardiovascular risk factors and risks for other chronic inflammatory diseases. (See Consider 8.)

CONSIDER 8

✅ Talk to your provider about getting a sleep study if you answer yes to some or all of these questions:

1. Have you been noted to have daytime sleepiness?
2. Do you snore?
3. Do you have uncontrolled blood pressure or a BMI (body mass index) of greater than 35?

What about Sleep Debt and Cancer?

Sleep deprivation has been associated with increased risk for cancers. Studies show a relationship of sleep to the hormone melatonin. Melatonin, along with promoting sleep, has been shown to inhibit cancer development and growth and improve immune function. It also has an antioxidant effect.[32]

Some believe that sleep disturbance leads to immune suppression, which results in cancer-promoting cytokines. These cytokines are molecules that help with cell-to-cell communication in immune responses and help mobilize cells to move to sites where there is inflammation. One study in Denmark showed a 1.5-fold increase in risk for primary breast cancer among women who worked mostly at night for at least six months. They also produced more cytokines, presumably because they didn't experience enough darkness. Without the darkness, they didn't produce enough melatonin to power their immune systems properly and cytokines developed.[33,34] It is hypothesized that melatonin is regulated by the retina in the back of the eyes, which recognizes light and darkness. Women who are blind and cannot detect light—and as a result their melatonin levels are not inhibited—have a 50 percent lower relative risk of breast cancer than women who can see light.[35]

Even weak light during nighttime decreases our melatonin production. Changing work hours isn't always something we can control, but reducing ambient light by turning off email, reading print books rather than reading on a tablet or other electronic device, and not watching TV at night can not only improve our sleep but may lower our risk of certain cancers as well.

Blue Light

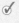tudies have looked at the role of electronics and brain wave chemistry at bedtime and its effect on melatonin. A 2014 study published in *The Proceedings of the National Academy of Sciences* showed that reading from an electronic book instead of a traditional book increased the time needed to fall asleep because of reduced drowsiness. Further, melatonin levels of those in the study were lower in the blood at night, and people were less alert in the morning than those who read a paper book.[36]

In preindustrial times, our cues for circadian rhythm were based on sunlight. The pineal gland in our brains releases melatonin rhythmically, with levels peaking during the dark period at night.[37] However, our use of alternative light sources sends signals to our retina, stimulating our photosensitive retinal ganglion cells, also called ipRGCs, which can detect ambient light information and signal our brains to cut back on melatonin production.[38] These cells have a crude ability to pick up light, so a night-light or a light placed far from us usually will not impact these changes. It is the brighter items—our electronics, lights on in rooms—that affect our melatonin levels. Also, it turns out that these cells are most sensitive to blue light, which is what most tablets emit.[39]

Mariana Figueiro of the Rensselaer Polytechnic Institute has done extensive research on these changes.[39] She also found out that blue light leads to a faster heart rate and causes EEG changes (brain wave changes), which show increased beta waves and correspond to increased alertness. You can avoid this by using a filter with your device, dimming the light (or switching it to night mode), or holding your device farther away from your eyes. (See Consider 9.)

CONSIDER 9

✓ You can decrease the alertness caused by your devices by using a filter with your device, dimming the light (or switching it to night mode), or holding your device farther away from your eyes.

Crazy Thought

We believe the one hour of productive work you think you get at the very end of the day is often negated by the sluggishness and decreased alertness you experience in the morning. We think we all should learn to shut down our electronics at least two hours before bedtime. We realize that in our global economy, there is always daylight in some part of the world, and some professions expect a 24/7 approach. However, if you look at it from a productivity perspective, the science shows that restful sleep leads to better performance and longevity. (See Consider 10.)

CONSIDER 10

Challenge yourself to turn off your electronics one to two hours prior to bedtime. Too much? OK, then start smaller and try increasing it in increments of 30 minutes.

Teens

One of our biggest concerns is the lack of sleep among teens. The circadian rhythm in teens is different from that of adults; they tend to be night owls, and their rhythms shift toward a melatonin surge later in the evening. They also are more sensitive to blue light than adults, which adds to the daytime drowsiness brought on by their early school schedules. The American Pediatric Association recommends 8.5 to 10 hours of sleep for teenagers, but fewer than 50 percent of American teens get that sleep. A University of Minnesota study showed that high schools that moved their start times to 8:30 a.m. noticed improved grades in school and achievement tests, better attendance rates, and reduced car accident rates. Other studies show that better sleep translates into better behavior and mood in adolescents.[40] (See Consider 11.)

CONSIDER 11

If our children are allowed to sleep without interruption, when would they naturally wake up?

Learning and Detoxification

How does sleep refresh us? Scientists have shown through animal trials that our brain cells can shrink during sleep, which allows for increase in interstitial space, or space between cells. They further observed that during this sleep time, the fluid between the cells and the cerebrospinal fluid, which bathes our nerve tissues, increases the rate of removal and clearance of proteins such as B amyloid and other neurotoxins (toxins for the brain). Their findings suggest that sleep, more than wakefulness, more effectively removes waste products or detoxifies our brains after a day of activity.

Barbara Oakley, PhD, a professor of engineering at Oakland University, teaches courses on learning and feels that sleep is critical to learning new material. She states, "This nightly house cleaning is part of what keeps your brain healthy. When you get too little sleep, the buildup of these toxic products is believed to explain why you cannot think very clearly." She highlights the role of sleep in learning and creativity in her book *A Mind for Numbers* and in her free online course called "Learning How to Learn."[41] She reports that falling asleep while thinking about difficult concepts can help cement the learning processes for new ideas and concepts. Examples of famous intellectuals who used sleep to formulate new ideas are Thomas Edison and Salvador Dali; both got into mindsets that were very relaxed and eventually they drifted off to sleep. Some historians believe they discovered new ways to approach their tough problems using this technique and were able to think of creative solutions when they awoke.

People often wear sleep deprivation as a badge of honor on their sleeves. Some correlate it with improved efficiency, and what they consider as excess sleep has at times been equated with laziness as well. However, if you look at it with productivity in mind, the science shows that restful sleep leads to better performance and longevity. In addition, research has shown that sleep deprivation increases our sympathetic overdrive, decreases healing, and reduces important hormones, such as growth hormone. Further, sleep deprivation impairs memory, leads to glucose imbalances, reduces our ability to detox, and leads to weight gain. Along with decreased reaction time, higher risk for accidents,

| FIGURE 4 | Sleep Hygiene* |

Practices that can help you get a good night's sleep:

- Exercise can promote good sleep but some people can have a hard time falling asleep when they exercise at night because of the endorphin—adrenalin release. And so exercise, but exercise early

- Avoid food too close to bedtime, especially if you have issues with heartburn

- Keep room dark during the night

- Try to get natural light during the day

- Switch off your electronics 1-2 hours before bed

*adapted from the National Sleep Foundation

inhibiting creativity, and worsening mood, sleep deprivation leaves you with much more than just being tired; sleep deprivation also increases your risk of chronic disease.

Not convinced? Why don't you sleep on it? (See figure 4.)

YOUR PRESCRIPTION

1. Try to work toward sleeping the goal allotment for your age. Add 15 minutes of sleep each week and build up. Whatever it is that's keeping you up can wait till morning

2. Avoid looking at your electronics for one to two hours prior to bed. Too hard? Start with 30 minutes

3. When you lie down and your mind is racing, start taking deep breaths. Focus on your breath. Take 10 deep breaths. Exhale twice as long as you inhale. Bet you won't make it to 10.

13

The Mind-Body Connection

Unleash the healing power of a calm mind

CASE 1: A 50-year-old male who was 100 pounds overweight, a photographer and videographer, came to our office. He had a history of knee pain, diabetes, and high cholesterol. Due to his knee pain and fatigue, he led a mostly sedentary life. Two years ago, he started a weekly Bikram yoga class in order to spend more time with his girlfriend. Bikram yoga is a type of yoga where poses are done under high heat and humidity to trigger a significant sweat response. He had difficulty staying in the class for the first few sessions due to the excessive heat. But in each class he did a little more. He stayed with the classes and noticed they gave him more energy and cleared his mind. He realized that he wanted to make better food choices, and as his muscle strength grew, he was able to increase activity outside the class. He then added cycling to his regimen.

Over the next two years, he lost 100 pounds and came off most of his pain medications, and his metabolic issues diminished. He continues to lead an active lifestyle. At present, he continues his yoga, along with the other cardiovascular exercises. Yoga makes him feel peaceful, he says, and improves his creativity. His arthritis is gone. His diabetes and high cholesterol have resolved.

CASE 2: A 50-year-old male executive came in for a physical exam. His travel and meeting schedule did not allow him to fast properly for blood work or show up for his appointment. He had to reschedule his visit three times in three months due to urgent conflicts. During the entire appointment, his phone vibrated with new texts and calls. It turned out his cardiovascular testing and fitness were normal, but his stress parameters on a questionnaire and adaptability to stress were very abnormal. Upon further questioning, he reported that he was feeling intense stress all of the time. His business was extremely successful, and he had an active, supportive family; however, he constantly worried about the next steps for his business. His health was stable at the time of his visit, but we wondered how he would do after five to ten years of this constant stress. We wondered what tools we could provide him to calm himself.

Does this sound like you or someone else you know, who multitasks all day? How many of us have been in a situation where we have had to add much more to our plates for several weeks or months? You look back and say to yourself, "How did I ever manage that?" Well, it was your acute stress response and adaptation. During such times, it's important to eat nutrient-rich foods with high levels of antioxidants and rest well to be able to sustain yourself. After it is over, you need a period to recharge yourself (activation of the parasympathetic nervous system). After using all the gas, we have to go to the refilling station. If we don't refill, recharge, and refresh, we break down just like our cars.

Our bodies break down too. But how do we reduce our stress? How do we learn to calm down? Sometimes this is easier said than done. Sometimes it is hard to shut off the stimuli and slow down, no question. But what if you had a tool to improve your sense of peace, reduce the dread and anxiety of the stress, lower the inflammation and oxidative stress, and improve restorative sleep before, during, and after the stress was over?

Mind/Body Techniques

When we were in medical school, we were told treatments for certain illnesses were lifestyle changes. Those changes were usually summed up as eating a good diet, exercising, and reducing stress. Ask most physicians, and they can't explain what "lifestyle changes" truly means because, the truth is, we aren't taught how to make those lifestyle changes in medical school. We know that sleep is important but weren't taught how to aid sleep. We know that exercise is important but weren't taught what exercises to give our patients. And we certainly were not taught techniques for reducing stress in medical school. We have learned these tools from personal experience, and then we started going back to the data. We now teach our patients how to decrease stress. These tools are often called mind/body techniques, and they encompass yoga, exercise postures, breathing techniques, and meditation. Studies show how such techniques help suppress sympathetic overdrive and increase the rest and recovery function of the parasympathetic nervous system.[1] These techniques help us refill our tanks.

What Is Yoga?

While many people think of yoga as just a series of postures, it is actually a combination of breathing exercises (pranayama),

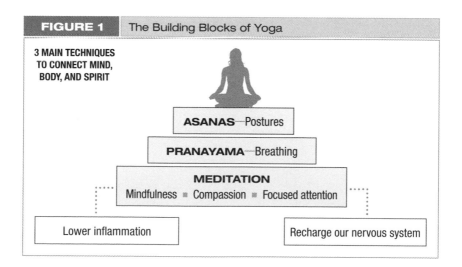

FIGURE 1 The Building Blocks of Yoga

3 MAIN TECHNIQUES TO CONNECT MIND, BODY, AND SPIRIT

ASANAS—Postures

PRANAYAMA—Breathing

MEDITATION
Mindfulness ▪ Compassion ▪ Focused attention

Lower inflammation

Recharge our nervous system

postures (asanas), and meditation together. (See figure 1 on the previous page.) The poses typically utilize isometrics, building muscles by holding a pose to cause muscle contraction while not bending at the joint as you would with free weights. The movement from one pose to another can provide a terrific cardiovascular workout.

Pranayama breathing utilizes diaphragmatic (big belly) breathing while varying the speed and duration of respiration and the lengths of inhalations and exhalations. The breath, especially while exhaling, is a very powerful tool for activating the parasympathetic nervous system. It can slow down both the heart and respiration rate. (See Consider 1). Yogic meditation retrains the mind to achieve a state of calm using focused attention, mindfulness, and compassion meditation. Focused attention allows for a concentration on breathing cycles, sound, or chants; its goal is to train the mind not to wander and focus on something singular, such as the breath. Mindfulness observes the current moment's experience, such as the breath, the sounds around us, and our thoughts, but noticing them without emotion. Guided meditation, when someone provides verbal instructions or suggestions, is also a form of mindfulness. Many people have found this form of practice to be a good way to begin. Guided meditation trains our minds to be more in the moment. Compassion meditation cultivates feelings of benevolence toward other people.[2] It often employs a repetitive phrase to foster feelings of universal good and is intended to decrease anxiety and burnout—especially useful for caregivers. (See Case 3.)

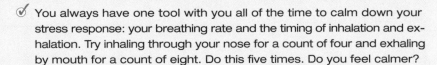

CONSIDER 1

☑ You always have one tool with you all of the time to calm down your stress response: your breathing rate and the timing of inhalation and exhalation. Try inhaling through your nose for a count of four and exhaling by mouth for a count of eight. Do this five times. Do you feel calmer?

CASE 3: Dr R: I used to see 25 people per day. Halfway through the day, I was completely wiped out, trying to give my patients full attention and empathy. I would have to force myself to take 20 minutes and meditate. I would come back feeling recharged and ready for the rest of the day. It has always amazed me how relaxing the mind can recharge the whole body.

History of Yoga

Yoga originated in the East. Yoga postures can be seen on artifacts dating back 5,000 years, and yoga is commented on in some of the earliest religious texts. In these references, yoga was seen as a tool to create harmony. Initially, it was meant for community wellness before it became an individual regimen. Highly spiritual leaders would guide people in ritual and ceremony to overcome the limitations of the mind. In these early texts, it was noted that yogic practice also included meditation. People would focus on the lotus pose that Buddha used in order to achieve enlightenment.

Over the centuries, the practice of yoga has transformed from being ceremonial and meditative to having an increased emphasis on fixed postures. In the nineteenth century, yoga was introduced in the West by Swami Vivekananda at the World Parliament of Religions in Chicago. His speech on Eastern tradition and yoga was received with a standing ovation. At the time, the focus of yoga was on health and vegetarianism. After this, more and more Eastern influence made its way to America. In 1920, Paramahansa Yogananda, author of *Autobiography of a Yogi* (which is a classic in spiritual literature), spoke at a religious conference in Boston.[3] This event triggered a fascination with the Eastern practice of using yogic postures as a health tool. By the 1960s, Maharishi Mahesh Yogi popularized Transcendental Meditation.

The Benefits of Yoga

In clinical practice, yoga is prescribed to help with sleep problems; stress, balance, or gait problems; and to assist with weight loss. Yoga can build muscle, improve memory, and reduce pain.[4,5] Done routinely, yoga arguably, comes closer than any other practice to a true antiaging routine. The term "antiaging," however, really is a misnomer. Goals of anti-aging are not to stop the aging process but rather to age gracefully, which includes being disease free and preserving vision, cognitive health, and body structure. (See Consider 2 on the next page.)

CONSIDER 2

☑ What are our goals as we age? Is it to fight the process of aging or is the goal really to age with grace and strength? We want to be disease free, have good vision, and preserve memory and body structure. Yoga has been shown to help decrease chronic illness, preserve memory, and maintain body structure.

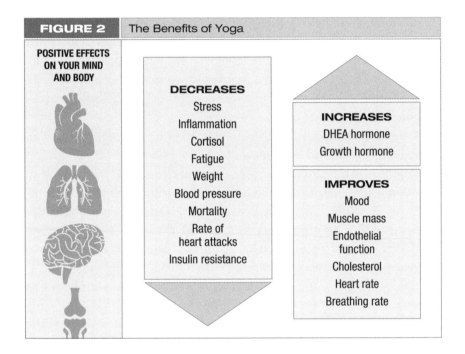

FIGURE 2 | The Benefits of Yoga

POSITIVE EFFECTS ON YOUR MIND AND BODY

DECREASES
Stress
Inflammation
Cortisol
Fatigue
Weight
Blood pressure
Mortality
Rate of heart attacks
Insulin resistance

INCREASES
DHEA hormone
Growth hormone

IMPROVES
Mood
Muscle mass
Endothelial function
Cholesterol
Heart rate
Breathing rate

Yoga, Inflammation, and Its Potential Role in Aging

The average lifespan around the world is increasing. The Centers for Disease Control (CDC) reports that life expectancy in the US is at a record high of 78.8 years for those born in 2012—females live for an average of 81.2 years and males live 76.4 years. As we age, the likelihood of contracting a chronic illness increases. With chronic illness, inflammation grows. We desperately need tools to help us age gracefully, preserve our minds and body structures, and improve our quality of life.

The goal of aging gracefully is to not live in a bubble. We cannot escape stress. It is part of life. But we can change the way in which our body perceives stress. Stress can be good because it raises our awareness. But it can also raise stress levels to a point where it causes anxiety and sleep disorders. Activation of the sympathetic nervous system during the alarm phase or period of acute stress can set up a cycle of high adrenaline, leading to higher levels of cortisol. When left unchecked, these elevated levels can cause multiple symptoms of stress and lead to chronic illness. However, most forms of yoga recharge us and lower cortisol surges.[6,7,8]

One study looked at female breast cancer survivors who had breast cancers staged between levels II and IV. Researchers found that regular yoga practice of 90 minutes done twice weekly for eight weeks resulted in lower levels of both morning cortisol and evening cortisol levels and better overall well-being and fatigue scores.[9] These cancer patients felt better when they did yoga, and their stress markers went down!

There are also studies showing that relaxation responses, such as yoga, meditation, and breathing, can enhance mitochondria, the energy powerhouse of cells, by impacting the genes that regulate the energy-producing reactions of our body.[10] Energy is created through formation of ATP (adenosine triphosphate). Relaxation response has been shown to increase ATP and, therefore, increase mitochondrial energy production. This makes us more effective at utilizing our supply of ATP and balancing demand. At the same time, these practices have been shown to decrease inflammation causing decreasing production of proteins (such as NF-KB) that turn on inflammation cascades in the body. Lower levels of NF-KB in immune cells have also been correlated with lower oxidative stress. These data suggest that yoga can positively affect energy, inflammation, and oxidative stress pathways, which are all implicated in chronic disease and aging.

One recent study linked loneliness in older adults to inflammation and showed that a mindfulness program reduces both inflammatory markers in the blood and feelings of loneliness.[11] (See Consider 3 on the next page.)

Caregivers who have the burden of providing care to the chronically ill also experience high levels of stress. Recall that stress triggers inflammation.[12] One study looked at the inflammatory markers of family members caring for parents with dementia. They found that those caregivers who meditated 12 minutes daily for eight weeks were able to decrease the inflammatory markers in their bodies. As people are living longer, there are many families providing care to the elderly. This finding reminds us that meditation is a great tool for calming stress and reducing inflammation in this caregiver population.[12]

CONSIDER 3

☑ Consider that here is another tool to decrease the inflammation in our blood!

Yoga and Hormone Balance

One of the most frustrating aspects of aging for both patients and physicians is hormone imbalance. Yoga has the ability to affect our hormone balance and directly address that stress response. More on this in a minute. First, let's talk about a few basics. Hormones are proteins in the body that communicate between different organs and tissues. They regulate most functions in the body, such as (but not limited to) digestion, metabolism, sleep, reproduction, and mood. Hormone imbalance and decline in most hormones are key factors in aging.

For example, dehydroepiandrosterone (DHEA) and growth hormone are naturally occurring hormones that decline as we age. DHEA has been linked to muscle mass, vitality, and cognitive health. Growth hormone, which is secreted from the pituitary gland of the brain, is linked to our ability to grow and heal. One study looked at the effects of regular yoga training for 12 weeks. Researchers observed that subjects who practiced yoga (using postures, breathing, and meditation) had higher levels of DHEA and growth hormone. The training utilized breathing practices, meditation techniques, and poses in various combinations over different time periods.[13] Yoga is an amazing way to naturally elevate hormones, especially as we age.

Adiponectin is a hormone generated by fat tissue. It is key to the metabolism of fat and glucose. Visceral fat, or belly fat, surrounds our internal organs. Excessive visceral fat is linked to an increase in inflammatory markers. Studies show yoga helps to reduce weight, improve muscle mass, and decrease blood pressure, along with reducing inflammatory markers. Yoga also increases adiponectin levels, which then regulate glucose and fat metabolism and assist with weight management.[14] (See figure 2 on page 144.)

Other studies find yoga helps to reduce hormones associated with polycystic ovary syndrome (PCOS). PCOS is a disorder where the balance between a woman's estrogen and testosterone becomes imbalanced. Women will have excess testosterone leading to irregular menstrual cycles, acne, excessive hair growth, insulin resistance, and infertility. Yoga has been shown to favorably impact glucose metabolism, lipids, and hormone balance that occur with PCOS. One study showed yoga was superior to exercise in lowering insulin resistance, which is a precursor to diabetes.[15]

Yoga and Cardiovascular Benefits

Stress is increasingly identified as a culprit in cardiovascular illness. The link is felt to be through the effects of cortisol and the sympathetic nervous system.[16] Stress appears to trigger endothelial dysfunction (inability of the blood vessels to dilate appropriately). Damage to the endothelium has been implicated in the formation of plaque. One study looked at healthy men who were given a mental stress test. Researchers found that after periods of mental stress, the men had endothelial dysfunction for up to four hours.[17] It is amazing to think that our stress can trigger heart disease. This further emphasizes the importance of having tools to decrease stress.

In another study, stress reduction techniques, such as yoga and meditation, were examined in 33 people both with and without heart disease. Participants meditated and did yoga for weeks. In the participants with cardiovascular disease, yoga and meditation improved endothelial function significantly.[18] Although this particular study did not find significant change in endothelial function in the individuals without heart disease, they did find a decrease in blood pressure, heart rate, and BMI (body mass index) in both the participants with and without heart disease.

Even with all of our current advances in knowledge about medications, procedures, and surgical interventions, cardiovascular disease still remains the leading cause of death in the US. Pioneers in lifestyle medicine, such as Dean Ornish, MD, realized more than 30 years ago that lifestyle changes, including stress reduction strategies such as yoga and meditation combined with dietary changes, can reduce risk factors for cardiac health. With these lifestyle changes, parameters that improved were cholesterol, endurance, work performance, and heart function.[19] More recently, the *European Journal of Clinical Cardiology* looked at more than 37 randomized controlled trials on asana-based yoga practice and found lower cardiovascular risk factors, such as lower BMI, systolic blood pressure, total cholesterol, and triglyceride and LDL levels. Higher HDL levels were also noted. They concluded that there is promising evidence for yoga's improving heart health.[20] In fact, when comparing participants who did yoga but no traditional cardiovascular exercise to those who did traditional exercise, the study showed there was no difference in their heart health. It suggests that yoga shows promise in improving cardiovascular health.

Yoga and Mood

As clinicians, we also like to give people the lifestyle tools they need to regulate mood issues. One mindfulness program initiated by Jon Kabat-Zinn, PhD, at the University of Massachusetts, entitled Mindfulness Based Stress Reduction (MBSR), has become quite popular. He has created an eight-week program that teaches mindfulness in a stepwise fashion. Kabat-Zinn's programs have been studied in research trials and have been found to deliver significant benefits, so that more than 250 hospitals worldwide use them as an adjunct to health care in a variety of areas.

MBSR has been used successfully to help people with irritable bowel syndrome (IBS), which has a significant stress component. There has always been a strong connection between mood and the gut. IBS is considered a functional illness because its symptoms (such as bloating, gas, and constipation alternating with diarrhea) relate to the gut's functions, but there are no structural, infectious, or microscopic changes in the gut. Often, these symptoms are triggered by emotion. It is a very common diagnosis with limited treatment options, which frustrates both patients and providers. However, in one study, the group who completed MBSR training showed a reduction in the severity of symptoms of IBS and the symptoms of stress, both of which were maintained at the six-month follow-up.[21] One of the most exciting studies recently published was conducted at Johns Hopkins University in 2014. This study reviewed more than 18,000 meditation studies over 47 different research trials and found that mindfulness programs improved levels of anxiety, depression, and pain.[22]

In areas where stress can play a large role in flares, such as with inflammatory bowel disease, research has shown that those people with the highest stress markers (measured by urinary cortisol) were the ones who reported better quality-of-life scores with mindfulness practice, even during their flares.[23] If we extrapolate from this, then mindfulness will have benefit in so many chronic illnesses.

Yoga, Learning, and Memory

Meditative techniques have been found to augment specific areas of the brain that relate to restfulness, but they also improve attention skills and reaction time to stimuli. These meditative techniques actually shrink areas of the brain involved with anxiety, rage, and low mood.[2] In addition, the most exciting aspect of meditation for us is that it builds up the gray matter in the front of the brain—a good thing. This is called the prefrontal cortex and is associated with working memory (or making new memories).

A study from Harvard University showed that parts of the nerve cell called axons, which transmit information to other cells, can increase in the brain of those who meditate.[24] Other studies have shown that meditative practices, such as restful waking (lying awake in the dark and focusing on breathing), facilitate auditory learning.[25] This means that just the practice of resting and focusing on being calm can improve the ability to learn through hearing. Further, meditation can increase the connections between cells which will increase memory, overall brain function, and resilience to stress.[24] In a time when the rates of Alzheimer's disease are exponentially increasing, this is very exciting information and could potentially help us with the war against brain thinning (atrophy) and memory loss. (See Consider 4.)

CONSIDER 4

✓ Yoga is another tool that will help your memory and your ability to combat stress, as well as improve overall brain function.

Yoga and Alignment

Yoga also incorporates a focus on posture and alignment. Poor posture and alignment have been linked to many medical disorders. Having a curved spine as a result of sitting for 8 to 10 hours per day has many detrimental effects, not only on stature. It also can be the source of pain issues and decreased energy and can play a role in other chronic disease states. Regarding chronic illness, prolonged sitting can cause our muscles to utilize insulin less effectively. This can directly lead to issues with glucose metabolism and eventually with insulin resistance and prediabetes. Prolonged sitting can also be associated with pain syndromes. Strained neck, carpal tunnel, shoulder pain, and lower back and hip pain can all arise from sitting. In an age when most of us sit—commuting to work and sitting in a car for two hours per day, then sitting at a desk for eight hours—our posture and alignment can suffer.

Normal alignment requires three curves of the spine, which contains 33 bones arranged as the cervical (C1–C7), thoracic (T1–T12), lumbar (L1–L5), and sacral (S1–S5) sections. (See figure 3 on page 151.) With good posture and a neutral spine, we have a slight cervical curve (anteriorly or toward the front of the body), thoracic curvature posteriorly, and lumbar curvature anteriorly. Sitting at a desk at work and typing for long periods can put a large strain on many different parts of this system. For instance, sitting at a desk causes forward protrusion of the neck, which can result in not only cervical or neck issues but also upper back and shoulder issues. The counterbalance is to keep the shoulders relaxed and the neck from leaning forward, while sitting with the pelvic muscles flexed and keeping the feet flat on the floor.

Sitting for long periods also causes tightening of the hip flexors and weakness in the gluteal and abdominal muscles. This can lead to stiffness and inflexibility and can impact our spinal discs. It also causes instability and increases the risk of falling. Yoga poses can combat these issues with their focus on lateral movement, extension of the spine, and balance. Imagine how good you feel when you do a light stretch after a prolonged period of sitting; now imagine what a daily practice with yoga could do for combating the stress on our bodies from our daily routines.

Diaphragmatic breathing, which is a form of breathing practiced during yoga, can utilize shoulder, thorax, and abdominal muscles more efficiently if done periodically during the work day. In fact, one meta-analysis showed an improvement in lung flow for people with chronic obstructive pulmonary disease (COPD) when they practiced yoga.[26] The mechanism is not clear, but it may involve relaxing the

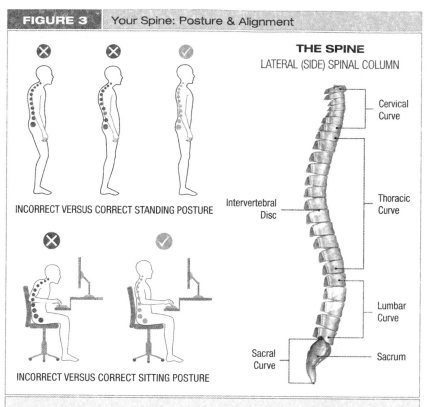

FIGURE 3 | Your Spine: Posture & Alignment

INCORRECT VERSUS CORRECT STANDING POSTURE

INCORRECT VERSUS CORRECT SITTING POSTURE

THE SPINE
LATERAL (SIDE) SPINAL COLUMN

Cervical Curve

Thoracic Curve

Intervertebral Disc

Lumbar Curve

Sacral Curve

Sacrum

With good posture and a neutral spine, we have a slight cervical curve (anteriorly or towards the front of the body), thoracic curvature posteriorly, and lumbar curvature anteriorly. Sitting at a desk causes forward protrusion of the neck, which can result in not only cervical or neck issues but also upper back and shoulder issues due to the trapezius muscle that connects them.

body, as well as improving muscle function. It also allows for a focus on neutral spinal alignment, which benefits air entry.

Many yoga poses, such as downward-facing dog or the cat and cow pose, work on the opposing muscles that are contracted while sitting all day. Adding stretches and yoga poses into your day or using a sit-stand desk can help protect against the adverse health effects caused by sitting eight hours a day. There are many websites available that summarize up-to-date research on the benefits of sit-stand desks.

Expert opinion and research have shown that prolonged sitting can have an effect on our response to insulin. *The Washington Post* ran an article several years ago showing the hazards of sitting on many organs in the body. The authors showed a decrease in appropriate insulin response after only one day of prolonged sitting.[27] Other studies show that yoga postures and meditation reduced fasting glucose and insulin levels, suggesting that the pancreas became more sensitive to glucose signals and did not have to work as hard. We can now consider using yoga to decrease our sugar levels.[28,29]

Yoga and Your Pelvic Floor

Women often experience difficulty with holding their urine at one time or another. This is called stress incontinence and can often be triggered by excessive impact, as happens with running, excess weight, and multiple pregnancies. Stress incontinence can also happen with hormone changes in menopause. Symptoms are frustrating for women who often have to urinate frequently and have small amounts of urine leakage when coughing, sneezing, laughing, or exercising.

Pelvic floor yoga (yoga that works on the muscles, ligaments, and nerves that support organs such as the bladder, uterus, rectum, and vagina) is a great tool for combating urinary incontinence. Our pelvic floor muscles are use-it-or-lose-it muscles. We need to work on them actively to maintain them. Kegel exercises are a type of pelvic floor workout that utilizes contractions of the pelvic floor muscles for 5 to 10 seconds at a time to mimic the cessation of urine flow. These work, but they need to be done several times each day. We recommend linking Kegel exercises to an activity that happens often in your day, such as receiving a phone call or sending an email. However, adding pelvic floor yoga takes Kegels to a new level. We have found pregnancy yoga tapes to be helpful for bladder strengthening. These exercises are simple and can be done sitting in a chair even when at work.

Types of Yogic Poses

There are numerous types of yoga, which can make starting a practice confusing and overwhelming. As you will see, however, any of the many yoga practices can offer incredible health benefits.

Yoga can be broken down into many different styles. One common style of yoga seen in the US is hatha yoga. Hatha yoga is an umbrella term for the practice that utilizes asanas or poses in combination with breathing techniques. Power yoga is a high-intensity style, popular in gyms, which focuses on flow from one pose to another and is primarily intended to build strength and flexibility. Iyengar, anusara, and viniyoga are other common styles that are slow-paced and focus on alignment. Kripalu yoga is a slow-movement style that emphasizes mind/body awareness. Kundalini yoga uses more meditation, chanting, and breathing along with poses.

A challenging type of yoga now commonly practiced in the United States is ashtanga yoga, which features constant movement and breathing techniques. Through movement, heat is generated, which is felt to be vital to yogic practice. Bikram yoga is another such yoga. Bikram yoga features 26 fixed postures, each repeated twice and performed in a room with 40 percent humidity, heated to more than 104° Fahrenheit. Practitioners often excessively sweat as they complete the postures. These higher intensity yoga styles are recommended for those who do not have active medical issues. As you can see, there are many types of yoga, making it easy to individualize a practice to fit each person's needs. (See figure 4.)

FIGURE 4	Numerous Types of Yoga	
STYLE	**INTENSITY**	**HIGHLIGHTS**
Hatha Yoga	Variable	Umbrella term for styles working with poses and breath
Power Yoga	High	Continuous sequence of poses
Iyengar/ Anusara Yoga	Medium	Emphasis on proper alignment
Kripalu Yoga	Low	Encourages mind/body awareness
Kundalini Yoga	Low/Medium	Encourages self empowerment; utilizes chanting, poses, and breath
Ashtanga Yoga	High	Series of scripted poses, create your own heat, focuses on rhythmic breathing
Bikram Yoga	High	Series of scripted poses in artificial heat

Yoga is a physical, mental, and spiritual discipline with a broad variety of schools, practices, and goals

A Unique Type of Yoga: Yoga Nidra

ur favorite type of yoga is called yoga nidra, which allows us to enter a state between wakefulness and sleep.[30] Yoga nidra is referred to as yogic sleep and is a practice in which you lie in savasana (corpse pose). You utilize breathing techniques, followed by periods where you focus on one body part at a time, then follow a guided meditation. It has been shown to induce alpha brain waves, which are associated with a relaxed mental state. Yoga nidra improves restful sleep but does not have to be done at night. It recharges the autonomic nervous system by improving the parasympathetic (rest and digest) component. It is an excellent tool for facilitating sleep when a person is aroused at night. (See Consider 5.)

CONSIDER 5

☑ Do you find that you have difficulty calming your racing mind when you wake up at night? Yoga nidra can be a great tool for this.

Transcendental Meditation

ranscendental Meditation (TM) is another specific form of mind/body intervention that has generated compelling data regarding cardiovascular medicine. It is a form of meditation that uses a mantra—a word or sound that has phonetic significance—in order to settle the mind. TM is a technique performed for 20 minutes twice a day. Some benefits are related to a drop in cortisol levels of up to 30 percent.[31,32] Studies show that a TM practice reduces sympathetic nervous system activation.[33] Lower cortisol and decreased sympathetic activation have shown benefit in areas such as cardiovascular disease. One study showed that TM reduced the risk of mortality, myocardial infarction (MI), and stroke in patients with a history of heart disease.[34] In fact, the American Heart Association recommends the use of TM for prevention and treatment of hypertension.[35]

Yoga and the Community

oga has been used in many high-risk communities with amazing results. The goal of these community programs has been to create resiliency in residents of high-risk areas and rehabilitation to those who have been imprisoned. Police inspector Kiran Bedi used mindfulness breathing techniques to rehabilitate hardened criminals in Tihar Jail, one of the largest complexes of prisons in India. Her successful program educating the inmates about anger, fear, and hatred and turning them into productive members of society earned her international recognition and world praise.[36] Currently, programs are being instituted in select prisons from Seattle to Washington, DC, in hopes of using it to reduce violence and crime.

Another example of the benefits of yoga in the community is seen through the Holistic Life Foundation in Baltimore, Maryland.[37] This foundation teaches meditation to teachers, parents, and children. The foundation began its work in areas of high risk, such as inner-city Baltimore, more than 10 years ago and has expanded to many other locations and demographic areas. It offers residency programs where instructors teach mindfulness to children, helping them to cope with chronic stress and anxiety.

Other leaders, such as Arianna Huffington, founder of *Huffington Post*, are trying to change corporate culture by suggesting that companies add a daily meditation practice in the workplace, starting at the CEO level. Hopefully this cultural mindset of working and feeling guilty about taking time to recharge ourselves with tools like meditation will diminish when we see how productive and pleasant the workplace can be when people are recharged.

The Multitasking Elephant in the Room—Are We Overdoing It?

One common real-life occurrence is how often Dr A cannot find her car when she returns to a parking lot after an errand. She is usually the one pressing her key alarm and listening for her car to respond. Most of the time when she enters a building from a parking lot, she is catching up on phone calls, emails, or texts and reviewing her overscheduled day. Does this sound familiar? Being more present at the task at hand would solve the problem. We often think such forgetfulness is a memory issue, but that is not completely true. Memory is not the problem. It is our lack of mindfulness—focusing on the moment and being present in the moment without letting distractions get in the way of the current moment.

Technology has changed our lives. The advent of smartphones, tablets, and other devices helps get us information quickly and stay connected to one another. We have a wealth of guidance at our fingertips. However, these high-tech toys also serve as distractions and cause us to be less mindful. The constant buzz of incoming texts and social media messages takes us away from our thoughts and tasks. Multitasking is a misnomer and suggests efficiency; a better label would be "rapid toggling between tasks." Bob Sullivan and Hugh Thompson, in their *New York Times* article "Brain, Interrupted," describe research done at Carnegie Mellon by Alessandro Acuisti, PhD.[38] Acuisti showed that an increase in interruptions results in 20 percent lower test scores. That multitasking and constant toggling between tasks worsens performance. We think we are being more efficient, but in the long run, our efficiency is less, and we actually perform poorly. It's also important to incorporate technology-free times into your day, so you can focus on family, relationships, and calming the mind. (See Consider 6.)

CONSIDER 6

☑ Have you noticed how often your phone dings during the day or during an hour? In response, how often do you stop what you are doing to check the message? Consider how disruptive that is to your focus.

For the person in case 2 at the beginning of the chapter, Dr. R did recommend he try to practice mindfulness—do things with a focus on the current task, and don't get sidetracked by cell phone calls or texts while he is working on a specific task. It worked wonders for him

Bottom Line: We need to take time to recover our bodies. Period. Plan for technology-free time, focus on getting restorative sleep with yoga nidra, and practice meditation at least five times a week. That could mean doing anything mindfully—staring at a candle for five minutes, ironing, swimming, or taking a yoga class. In the end, it does not matter which type of activity it is; it's how often you do it that counts. Make mindfulness a daily practice. Just take a deep diaphragmatic breath, and swan dive into it!

YOUR PRESCRIPTION

1. Whatever method of yoga or meditation you decide to do, do it every day.

2. Learn deep breathing techniques.

3. Make technology-free time every day.

4. Focus on each task individually and avoid multitasking.

14

The Euphoria
of Exercise

Movement to reverse the damage of a sedentary lifestyle

CASE: One of Dr. R's patients is a 36-year-old woman who came to the office with symptoms of excessive sweating. The symptoms started more than three months prior; she would sweat all over her body and at inappropriate times. She also had been experiencing significant diarrhea. She had been treated for depression in the past and had been taking an antidepressant called duloxetine. She denied any change in her stress level or in the dose of her medication. Otherwise, she had been feeling well in terms of energy and stamina. In fact, she reported she had been exercising more and was training for a half marathon. Her symptoms worried her, and she wanted to rule out cancer.

Her initial testing and chest X-ray were all normal. Dr. R thought that perhaps her medication was creating side effects. This possibility surprised the patient as she had been taking the duloxetine for five years; she couldn't understand why it suddenly could have an adverse effect after taking it consistently for so long. Dr. R believed that her recent exercise surge was raising the levels of neurotransmitters (chemical "messengers" in the brain that are responsible for good mood). As a result, her dose had become too high for her. While she felt a good deal of anxiety about this possibility, the patient ultimately agreed to taper the dose, and her symptoms resolved without any rebound in her depression. As it turned out, the high dose of duloxetine was competing with the natural effects of running. Her sweating and other symptoms improved significantly after Dr. R cut the amount of antidepressant she took daily. She continued to run and felt great.

Exercise is defined as any physical activity done for a certain purpose. It is a regular, repeated activity that improves our physical fitness. For centuries, wellness advocates have promoted exercise as a way to boost health and avoid chronic illness. People who exercise can feel their heart rates increase, their muscles get stronger, and their speed increase. They have more power, agility, balance, and coordination.

But those physical improvements aren't the only reasons to exercise. Deliberate movement also improves our reaction time. We sweat, which drives out toxins from our bodies. Exercise also creates a feeling of euphoria and a sense of happiness; it gives us added energy, and it improves our quality of life, and our ability to think more clearly.[1,2]

Physiologic parameters also improve with exercise. We see improvements in endurance, strength, and flexibility, and better body composition (muscle to fat ratios). Exercise brings healthy changes to blood sugar levels, cholesterol, and metabolism. It lowers our risk of heart disease, stroke, type 2 diabetes, and certain types of cancers, such as breast and colon. Studies have even shown that death from all causes can be delayed by regular physical activity.[3]

How Much Exercise Is the Right Amount?

In 2007, the American Heart Association and the American College of Sports Medicine released guidelines to help both physicians and patients decide which activities people should undertake, and how much they should do each week, in order to achieve their goals. Recommendations for overall activity will be discussed in this chapter, but specific advice for goals such as weight loss, faster speed or athletic performance, or cardiovascular retraining should be personalized with the help of a physician. Generally speaking, the American Heart Association recommends at least 150 minutes of moderate exercise per week, which can be broken down into 30- to 60-minute sessions, five days per week. The guidelines recommend increasing intensity and frequency over time for maximum benefit.[4]

We often measure exercise intensity by the concept of metabolic equivalents of task (MET) per week. A MET is a measure of the energy expenditure of a physical activity. It is used to gauge the intensity of that activity. As we exercise, we need more air so we can get oxygen into our bloodstream and into our muscles. METs represent the oxygen uptake required relative to rest. For example, six METS means the oxygen required is six times what is needed when at rest. One MET is what occurs when quietly sitting, and three METs is equal to three times the energy of sitting. Twenty-three METs is equivalent to running a mile in 4.17 minutes. METs are calculated in a sample population. They are based on the average person but vary based on age and conditioning. For instance, a person who is 40 years old and has a high fitness level can walk at a pace of three to four miles per hour, which is equal to three METs for him or her, but for a 70-year-old man, that level would be considered more vigorous exercise and is closer to six to seven METS. METs give us general guidelines to assess a person's exercise capacity. Overall, moderate intensity exercise is considered exercise that results in three to six METs. Examples of such exercise are walking at a brisk pace at three to 4.5 miles per hour, hiking, roller skating, cycling at five to nine miles per hour, water aerobics, and carrying your clubs during a round of golf. Figure 1 on the next page can serve as a reasonable guideline.[5]

Population studies looking at both men and women have shown that when they exercised at a workload of three to 5.9 METs (moderate activity) for 150 minutes per week, there was a significantly decreased risk of heart disease and mortality.[6,7,8,9,10] Further studies show that when a sedentary lifestyle is broken up by bursts of activity, the risk of chronic illness is reduced.[11]

Current State of Affairs: The Coach Potato

The standards written by the American Heart Association and American College of Sports Medicine have been supported by numerous trials. However, society as a whole has had trouble following them. Overall, we are fairly sedentary. We sit behind our desks for eight hours a day, sit in our cars with long commute times, and watch TV or sit in front of the computer in the evenings before bed. People often say they don't have time or are too tired to exercise after a long day at work.

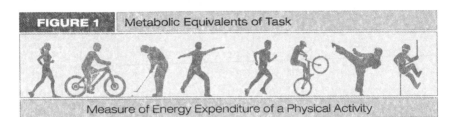

FIGURE 1   Metabolic Equivalents of Task

Measure of Energy Expenditure of a Physical Activity

MODERATE ACTIVITY (3.0 to 6.0 METs)

WALKING (MODERATE)

At a brisk pace of 3 to 4.5 mph on a level surface inside or outside, such as

- Walking to class, work, or the store
- Walking for pleasure
- Walking the dog
- Walking as a break from work
- Walking downstairs or down a hill

GENERAL HOME EXERCISES
(LIGHT OR MODERATE EFFORT)

- Getting up and down from the floor
- Trampoline jumping
- Stair climber
- Rowing machine

ACTIVITIES (MODERATE)

- Bicycling 5-9 mph, level terrain, few hills
- Stationary bicycling—moderate effort
- Racewalking—less than 5 mph
- Hiking
- Roller skating
- Aerobic dancing—high impact
- Water aerobics

SPORTS (MODERATE)

- Golf—walking with caddy
- Tennis (doubles)
- Badminton

VIGOROUS ACTIVITY (3.0 To 6.0 METs)

WALKING, JOGGING

- Race and aerobic walking—5 mph
- Jogging or running
- Wheeling your wheelchair
- Walking and climbing briskly up a hill
- Backpacking

BICYCLING

- Bicycling more than 10 mph or uphill
- Stationary bicycling—vigorous effort

EXERCISES (VIGOROUS)

- Calisthenics—push-ups, pull-ups,
- Jumping jacks
- Water jogging
- Stair climber machine—fast pace
- Rowing machine
- Arm cycling machine

ACTIVITIES (VIGOROUS)

- Roller skating—brisk pace
- Aerobics: step and dancing
- Karate, judo, tae kwon do, jujitsu
- Mountain rock climbing, rappelling

SPORTS (VIGOROUS)

- Tennis
- Basketball
- Swimming laps
- Surf boarding

With our sedentary lifestyle, obesity rates have risen. Current data from the Center for Disease Control and Prevention show that the US obesity rate reached 42.4 percent in 2017–2018.[12] Research shows that a sedentary lifestyle directly increases risk of coronary heart disease and depression, increases waist circumference, elevates blood pressure, worsens lipid profiles, and increases biomarkers, such as glucose and insulin (which can be precursors to diabetes).[13,14,15]

While a sedentary life can increase our risk of chronic illness, we also know that small increases in physical activity can reduce our risk of heart disease, stroke, type 2 diabetes, and certain cancers.[16] Small increases in movement can reduce mortality from all causes by 20 to 30 percent.[17] Any amount of exercise will help you live longer. Small changes, such as taking walking breaks during work, doing regular stretches, or increasing steps per day even by 2,000 steps, can help reduce our risk of serious illness.[18,19] As physicians, we recommend increasing exercise capacity because we know the substance called nitric oxide, which dilates our blood vessels, will build over time with continued exercise.[24] Exercise not only helps healthy blood vessels dilate but will ultimately help dilate thin, restricted vessels—and, over time, angina will diminish.[25,26] Exercise, however, should be done with caution and only after consultation with your physician. Further, we know that increasing nitric oxide can help prevent platelet aggregation (or platelet clumping), thus reducing the rate of plaque formation in your arteries.[27]

As we become more active, however, we need to move more to achieve benefit. The minimum at that point is not enough. Exercise has to reach a certain level of intensity, which is unique to each individual's fitness level and health status. If the exercise does not tax the body enough, the changes won't be as noticeable.

Of note, there is a phenomenon termed the "active couch potato." That term applies to the many of us out there who satisfy the 150 minutes of moderate exercise per week, but then the remainder of the time, we sit. Unfortunately, there is data coming out to suggest that even though we exercise, it is not okay to be sedentary the remaining time and that there are metabolic consequences to this behavior.[20] These studies were done on people who were spending excessive time watching television, but their results would apply to anyone who sits at a desk job and has long commuting times. Changes such as a sit-stand desk and activity during the day at work are of significant benefit. Think about the walk at lunch break, climbing stairs instead of using the elevator, and walking to and from work. We also have to minimize our screen time in the evenings to keep from having a couch potato persona. Consider cutting back on television, computer, and tablet time at the end of the day, and go for a nice evening walk. (See Consider 1.)

CONSIDER 1

Even though we cannot change our work or commute times, there are things we can change.

- ✓ Take the stairs instead of the elevator at work.
- ✓ Park farther away from the entrance to work.
- ✓ Decrease screen time.
- ✓ Go for a walk during lunch.

Exercise Does Not Always Equal Weight Loss

The American College of Sports Medicine recommends a range of 150 to 400 kilocalories of energy expenditure per day, a kilocalorie being what we commonly think of as a calorie. The term can be used to quantitate how much energy from food you take in or how much energy you burn. The amount of calories a person will lose is highly variable. Calories burned depends on your body height and weight, as well as the length and intensity of the exercise. For instance, a 160-pound man burns about 292 calories during one hour of cycling. The same size person will burn 402 calories during one hour of water aerobics. They will also burn 314 calories playing an hour of golf and carrying their golf clubs.[21] However, if a person is double that weight, the same activity will cause a significantly higher calorie loss. The larger you are, the more effort is required to move, and, therefore, more calories are lost. For example, a 160-pound person walking at a pace of 3.5 miles per hour (mph) can burn 314 calories in an hour, whereas someone who weighs 240 pounds burns 469 calories during that same hour.[22] (See figure 2 on the next page.)

Not all exercise will cause weight loss, however. Weight loss is based on so many factors: how much and what we eat and drink, how much we sleep, and what our hormone balance is. Weight loss to some extent is dictated by supply versus demand. In order to lose weight, the amount

FIGURE 2	Calories Burned (based on body weight and activity of one hour duration)	
	CALORIES BURNED	
PHYSICAL ACTIVITY	160 LB PERSON	240 LB PERSON
Running 5mph	606	905
High Impact Aerobics	533	796
Swimming Laps moderate	423	632
Water Aerobics	402	600
Low Impact Aerobics	365	545
Elliptical Trainer moderate effort	365	545
Golf with carrying clubs	314	469
Walking 2mph	204	305

*adapted from the mayoclinic.org

we take in must be less than what we lose through movement. Often, after initial quick weight loss, people plateau. Our bodies will then need more intense exercise to increase their calorie-burn rate. Sometimes increasing intensity is as easy as walking for an extra 10 minutes or adding weights while you walk. It is amazing how these small changes make huge differences.

The Biochemistry of Exercise

When we look at exercise, we see it in terms of metabolic fitness, which is what happens to the body on a cellular and hormonal level. Metabolic fitness can be divided into aerobic (with oxygen) and anaerobic (without oxygen). Both cause the heart rate to increase but have a very different role in maintaining health.

Exercise creates a physical stress that creates more demands on your body for oxygen, blood flow, and nutrients, and requires more energy production from your muscles to sustain activity. Increased activity creates a greater demand for oxygen. When we exercise, our cells use a form of energy called ATP (adenosine triphosphate). During exercise, our bodies use glucose (sugar) and fat to make this energy so we can keep going. We metabolize sugar or fat based on whether oxygen is present in our system or not.

At the beginning of an exercise session, we are primarily doing aerobic fitness because we have adequate oxygen to perform the required tasks at the beginning of our routines. Our heart rates increase to bring oxygenated blood to the muscles we are using. With oxygen, our bodies break down fat to make ATP so that our bodies can work more effectively. Although glucose is also being used in aerobic exercise, the primary source of energy is fat. For this reason, people often call aerobic fitness the fat-burn stage of exercise. (See figure 3.)

As we do more endurance work, our muscles demand oxygen and nutrients and run out of oxygen. We breathe faster to bring in more oxygen, and our heart rates go up to get the oxygen to the muscles that need it. Over time, however, we cannot get enough oxygen to the muscles that require it. Our muscle cells then shift to working without oxygen (anaerobic metabolism). Without oxygen, the body does not break down fat. It transitions to using glucose as the primary source of fuel for energy. When we use glucose without oxygen, lactic acid is the by-product. Lactic acid

---

FIGURE 3   Aerobic versus Anaerobic Metabolism

AEROBIC EXERCISE	ANAEROBIC EXERCISE
▪ Utilizes oxygen	▪ Without oxygen
▪ More efficient—releases more energy	▪ Less efficient—releases less energy
▪ Able to sustain for long periods	▪ More for high intensity
▪ Utilizes more fat more than glucose	▪ Utilizes glucose
▪ By products are CO_2, water and energy	▪ Creates lactic acid which can cause muscle fatigue
▪ Works at heart rates under 70% max HR	▪ Works at heart rates over 80% of max HR
▪ Can talk through	▪ Unable to talk through, feels uncomfortable
▪ Endurance workouts	▪ High intensity interval training, strength training with weights

Aerobic metabolism is when our muscles have adequate oxygen in them. Typically it occurs at the beginning of our exercise routine. Based on the intensity of our workout, aerobic metabolism can continue as long as our heart rates stay in the aerobic zone. As intensity and duration pick up, our muscles become depleted of oxygen and the body changes to anaerobic metabolism. It is then the muscles find other sources of energy, i.e. glucose. The byproduct of this metabolism is lactic acid which makes our muscles sore after workouts.

in our muscles is what makes them ache after a good workout. To help clear away the lactic acid, we activate our sympathetic nervous system (our fight-or-flight response) with the neurotransmitter norepinephrine (also called adrenaline). This allows our heart rate and blood pressure to further elevate and help bring more oxygen supply to our muscles.

This process of activating the nervous system is a form of stress. Exercise, though, is initially *eustress* because the increases in heart rate and blood pressure allow our oxygen supply to keep up with demand. The increase in heart rate also helps bring more oxygen to the tired muscles and aid in removing lactic acid. If we continue exercising, we accumulate even more lactic acid and speed up our heart rate even more. Eventually, based on our fitness levels, the muscles fatigue and we stop exercising.

Exercising beyond our fitness level can become a *distress*. We can become unbalanced and overwork our sympathetic nervous system. There is more adrenaline and the heart rate stays higher. Over time, this can cause injury and symptoms of overtraining, which can tax our immune systems.[23] Overdoing exercise will initially look like excessive muscle soreness and fatigue. With chronic imbalance, we start experiencing difficulty sleeping, recurrent illnesses and infections, mood disorders, and immune dysregulation. The immune system doesn't work as well. This is why it's important to build up slowly to an optimal fitness level.

While blood flow to the muscles and heart increases during exercise, exercise also increases blood flow to the skin, which helps dissipate the heat of muscle activity. However, because of this sympathetic overdrive, the blood vessels to other nonessential organs constrict to conserve resources. That is why if we eat and then exercise too soon afterward, we experience cramps. The body has pulled its blood flow away from the stomach to focus on movement and will only be allowed to fully metabolize that food when the parasympathetic is activated and recovery begins. In general, it's advisable not to eat heavy foods up to one hour prior to exercise.

It's Not All About the Workout: Making Time to Refuel

Positive structural and functional changes in the body occur with exercise and allow the body to adapt to increased demands. These adaptations occur during recovery. The body needs time to remove waste from cells, allow for the generation of new muscle, and form the necessary factors for generating energy production.[28] There needs to be time between workouts to allow for this process to occur. Especially when first starting an exercise program, it is advisable to allow one day between workouts of similar muscle groups. For instance, if we go for a run one day, the next day we should take up another activity. We should swim, do a cross-training or core exercise, or play tennis, for instance. Taking breaks between workouts allows the body to build up nutrients for the next workout and also to recover from the small injuries on a microscopic level that occur during exercise. Along with appropriate time between workouts, other factors such as balanced nutrition, proper hydration, and avoidance of extreme temperature can affect recovery.

There is some debate about the right carbohydrate-to-protein ratio and amounts of carbohydrate and protein to eat before, during, and after workouts. Dietary intake needs to be tailored to the intensity and type of workout. For example, intake of carbohydrates within two hours after a high-endurance workout, such as a marathon, is recommended to replace lost stores. Certain essential amino acids (called branched-chain), which are building blocks for protein, are helpful after a workout to help build new muscle.[29] We can get these amino acids from beans, lentils, pumpkin seeds, brazil nuts, walnuts, and cashews.[30] Remember, we need to take the time to restore balance in light of all the changes that happen after significant exercise. (See figure 4.)

If this time and support is not allotted, fatigue and muscle soreness can set in. If the body continues to be stressed, performance can fall, and you can develop an *overreaching syndrome*. The fatigue and muscle soreness that happens with overreaching syndrome can last from two weeks to two months, depending on the severity. Additional symptoms can be insomnia, increased immune dysfunction, and worsening allergies. It is felt that we are susceptible to this imbalance because of lower glycogen stores, decreased branched-chain amino acids, increased oxidative stress, and increased stress on the hormone and immune system. Adding periods of rest between workouts, taking supportive nutrients, and staying hydrated usually resolve this issue.[31]

If we don't heal overreaching syndrome, we can worsen the imbalance and develop a syndrome of *overtraining*. Overtraining exhibits as decreased physical performance, less interest in training, elevated resting heart rate, and poor concentration. With overtraining, we also see mood alterations, loss of appetite, and increased susceptibility to

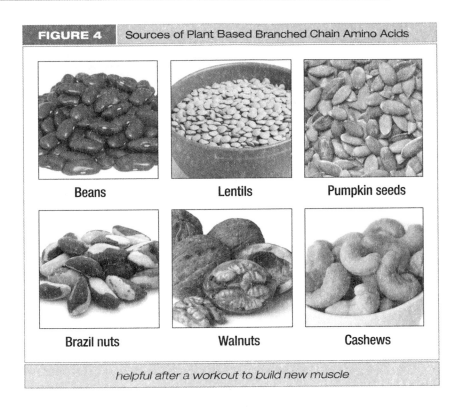

FIGURE 4 | Sources of Plant Based Branched Chain Amino Acids

Beans

Lentils

Pumpkin seeds

Brazil nuts

Walnuts

Cashews

helpful after a workout to build new muscle

injuries. This can last from eight weeks to three months even with rest.[31] Although rare, this spectrum of overreaching and overtraining syndrome is not just for the highly trained athlete. It can happen to those who do high-level physical activity in bursts, and their bodies have not been prepared for that intensity of exercise. In this situation, adaptation is markedly impaired and homeostasis is disturbed. This is why starting with a low-intensity exercise program and going slowly is a good idea; taking adequate rest between sessions can also help prevent these detrimental changes. (See figure 5 on the next page.)

Aerobic Versus Anaerobic Workouts

et's talk more about the difference between aerobic and anaerobic workouts. During times of rest and low-to-moderate levels of exercise (aerobic workouts), we don't produce lactic acid.[32] Usually, you can talk during this type of workout. It is highly efficient at producing energy for metabolism.

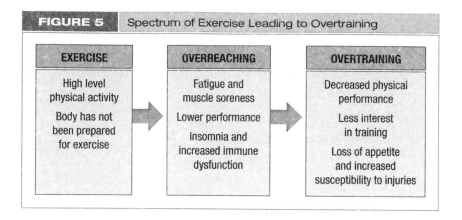

FIGURE 5 — Spectrum of Exercise Leading to Overtraining

EXERCISE	OVERREACHING	OVERTRAINING
High level physical activity Body has not been prepared for exercise	Fatigue and muscle soreness Lower performance Insomnia and increased immune dysfunction	Decreased physical performance Less interest in training Loss of appetite and increased susceptibility to injuries

Training is important to help increase the time we spend burning fat (aerobic) instead of glucose (anaerobic). Improved fitness leads to more efficient use of resources and better energy utilization.

A quick way to tell if you are entering the anaerobic phase is to watch your breathing. When breathing gets more labored (when you cannot talk during exercise), it usually means lactic acid is accumulating. The body is going into the anaerobic phase and is trying to release CO_2 and get more oxygen. The average shift to anaerobic metabolism occurs at about 85 percent of a person's maximum predicted heart rate (MPHR). Maximum predicted heart rate is determined by the number 220 minus your age. (See figure 6.) Getting up to 50 to 80 percent of your maximum heart rate is better for burning fat, but getting your

FIGURE 6 — The Average Shift to Anaerobic Metabolism

AGE	85% OF MPHR	
20 years old	170 heart rate	Maximum predicted heart rate = 220−age
30	162	
40	153	Most people shift to anaerobic metabolism at 85% of their maximum predicted heart rate
50	145	
60	136	
70	128	
80	119	

heart above 85 percent of your max heart rate can be better for an endurance workout. Many factors, such as your level of training, your fitness level, and what nutrient resources you have available, impact your transition from aerobic to anaerobic.

A gradual increase in intensity will facilitate better tolerance and make it easier to reach higher aerobic zones. It is important to discuss the safety of participating in activities that require endurance with your health-care provider, since the longer and more intense the workouts, the more your heart is taxed.

Swimming

An incredible exercise that we have learned to love is swimming. Swimming is the fourth most popular sports activity and is an excellent tool for endurance and resistance. It is often preferred by those who have chronic muscle or joint pain.[33] Studies have shown that in people with rheumatoid arthritis and osteoarthritis, swimming improves the joints without worsening symptoms.[34,35] This benefit can lead to better endurance in those who have other chronic medical problems as well.

Resistance Exercise

Resistance exercise is also called strength training. It focuses on building muscle and bone strength and increases metabolism.[36] The American Heart Association recommends that two sessions of muscle-strengthening activity be added on alternating days to our aerobic workouts.[4] One type of resistance is isotonic exercises. With isotonic exercises, the goal is to work on contracting the muscle by moving the joint and changing the muscle's length. Free weight lifting is an example of isotonic strength training. Lifting weights is a great way to build tone and bulk in muscle. The other type of resistance exercise is isometric exercise. With isometric exercise, the focus is contraction of the muscle without changing the joint angle or the muscle length. An example of this is using one's own body weight in a fixed position with weights or with yoga and core exercise. One of our favorite isometric exercises is the plank. (See figure 7 on the next page.)

Isometric exercises have therapeutic benefit because they can be done on immobilized limbs, since the joint doesn't need to move. They

FIGURE 7	Isotonic vs. Isometric

ISOTONIC	ISOMETRIC
Contracting the muscle by moving the joint and changing the muscle length	Contracting the muscle without changing the joint angle or muscle length
■ Weight lifting	■ Planks
■ Pull ups	■ Holding a squat
■ Sit ups	■ Fixed yoga poses

Two types of resistance exercise
or strength training—
focusing on building muscle/bone strength,
and increasing metabolism.

are of great benefit for older people because the exercises can be done in a seated position with very little space (in a cubicle or wheelchair).[37] Working on contracting muscles, such as the pelvic floor and gluteal and abdominal muscles, for fixed periods can add up, even when you do them for a few minutes at a time, several times a day during an eight-hour workday.

Benefits of Conditioning

As the body trains, it becomes more conditioned. Conditioning refers to a state where the cardiovascular system adapts to the increased requirements and demands of exercise and allows the heart to work more efficiently. There is more stroke volume (amount of blood per heartbeat) and increased output from the heart. With training, the capacity of the cells increases, and cells are able to deliver more oxygen to the rest of the body. As we train, our heart rates go down and resting blood pressure decreases. In addition, the energy producers of our cells, the mitochondria, have been found to increase in number with training.[38] With increased mitochondria, we become more energy efficient.

People often ask which type of cardiovascular exercise is best. The answer is that they are all good. Any exercise that helps us build muscles over time and condition our bodies is good. It is very important to vary workouts and not just focus on aerobic workouts alone.

Hormones

There is interplay between exercise and hormones. With moderate and intense exercise, cortisol levels increase. Cortisol can inhibit muscle growth and repair and can adversely affect our coordination.[28] Cortisol will increase in both fit and unfit individuals with exercise, but the levels are higher in an unfit individual. The amount of cortisol rise decreases as fitness increases.[39]

Anabolic hormones (hormones that build muscle) also rise with exercise. Testosterone, which is considered an anabolic hormone, can help build muscle and support red cells that carry oxygen. Resistance exercise and short-term intense interval exercise have shown to elevate testosterone levels.[40] Losing weight with exercise, especially abdominal fat, raises testosterone levels as well. Higher testosterone levels also help with recovery. Because of their higher testosterone levels, males can recover faster than females.[28]

Another anabolic hormone is growth hormone. Growth hormone increases muscle size and total body water content. It not only decreases body fat but also changes the distribution of body fat. Growth hormone levels increase with the intensity and duration of the workout. Moderate prolonged exercise can increase growth hormone levels tenfold. Data suggests that growth hormone is more associated with peak intensity of exercise than the total workout. Therefore, higher levels of the hormone are associated with higher intensity.[41]

Both testosterone and growth hormone can be regenerative due to their positive effects on muscle and how they aid in recovery. In cold temperatures, however, both hormones are inhibited, and, as a result, recovery time increases. In addition, as we age, both testosterone and human growth hormone decrease. Exercise, then, is a pleasant, natural way to boost both hormones.

How Does Exercise Affect Body Composition?

A combination of aerobic exercise and resistance exercise can impact cardiovascular health and can improve body composition. Exercise can increase muscle mass and decrease fat percentage, which can be key in managing inflammation and has a direct impact on our immune system.[42] As we discussed, inflammation has a strong

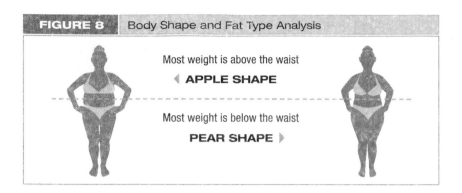

FIGURE 8   Body Shape and Fat Type Analysis

Most weight is above the waist
◀ **APPLE SHAPE**

Most weight is below the waist
PEAR SHAPE ▶

connection to many chronic disease states, such as diabetes, hypertension, coronary artery disease, and cancers.

There are two classic body types, based on both visceral fat (pro-inflammatory fat that surrounds our organs) and subcutaneous fat (which sits right under the skin). One body type is the pear shape, characterized by subcutaneous fat accumulation around the hips and buttocks. This fat is less of concern to one's health. Distribution of fat around the waist (leading to an apple shape) is more concerning because it is composed of both visceral and subcutaneous fat (See figure 8.)[42] Research shows that visceral fat can produce inflammatory cytokines (inflammatory chemicals) that alert our bodies to the presence of something foreign. Other proteins secreted by these fat cells directly result in insulin resistance, elevated blood pressure, altered clotting, and alterations in fatty acid metabolism.[43]

Visceral fat also affects our hormonal balance. For example, adrenal hormones, such as testosterone, can be converted to estrogen in our fat cells. Higher levels of estrogen have been linked to increased risk of postmenopausal breast cancer. There is also an increased conversion from inactive cortisone to active cortisol in our visceral fat. Active cortisol promotes more fat accumulation, which leads to increasing weight gain that can also propagate further hormone imbalance.[44] The good news is visceral fat is more affected by lifestyle changes than subcutaneous fat. By lifestyle changes, we mean that moderately intense activity along with dietary adjustments more effectively reduces visceral fat than subcutaneous fat.[45] Increasing nutrient-rich foods and cutting back on calorie-dense foods can be a great place to start. In fact, when vigorous exercise is a regular regimen, it's possible to lose adipose (fatty) tissue without losing weight because you're building lean muscle mass.[46,47]

Several studies have shown that stress is a major contributor to visceral fat and an altered cortisol response.[48] Cortisol is the hormone secreted by our adrenal gland when we are stressed. We see higher levels of cortisol in people who have stress related to their health, job, or schoolwork.[49] In some studies, the stress response has been shown to promote selective visceral fat accumulation and increased insulin resistance.[50] This shows us that stress or cortisol can promote abdominal fat.

Therefore, when you ask, "How do I lose my gut?," there is no easy answer. What we can tell you is to start with a nutrient-rich food plan and combine stress reduction with a balanced workout, including cardiovascular exercise, resistance, balance, and stretching. Sometimes working out *less* intensely can lower the stress response and improve abdominal fat. (See Consider 2.)

CONSIDER 2

The scale can be misleading when you are doing an exercise program. Often with good lifestyle changes, the scale does not change, but you will see changes such as loss of inches in the waist and hips.

CLINICAL CASE 1: The patient is an avid biker riding over 100 miles per week along with other high-intensity workouts per week. She changed her diet to help her prediabetes and was still struggling to lower her fat percentage and lose weight. She had a hamstring injury and could not maintain her high-intensity workouts; she finally took up yoga and lower intensity workouts. Within a few weeks, she noticed her waist size decrease and her weight reduced by eight pounds. She felt more energy as well.

HELPFUL TIP: High-intensity workouts can become stressful. They need to be balanced with lower intensity workouts. Yoga and Pilates are great choices.

CLINICAL CASE 2: The patient had a sedentary lifestyle and started walking 10,000 steps per day around her building. Along with dietary changes, she lost 15 pounds in six weeks, but then the weight loss stopped. Her body needed more cardiovascular exercise—walking was no longer enough. She then added three days of interval training weekly and continued to see weight loss of one pound per week.

TAKE HOME: Continue to challenge your body with varying workouts.

Brown Adipose Fat

I t is interesting to note that not all body fat is bad for health. Unlike white fat, brown adipose tissue (BAT) is a type of fat that boosts metabolic rate. This rate indicates how much energy we utilize when we're at rest. BAT fat is found in higher amounts in infants and decreases with age. The term "brown" comes from its high content of mitochondria, the energy producers in our cells. Studies have shown that when brown adipose fat is transplanted into mice, the recipient mice have improved glucose tolerance, increased insulin sensitivity, lower body weight, and reduced fat mass.[51] Researchers publishing in the journal *Nature* in 2012 showed that moderate exercise can transform white adipose tissue into brown adipose tissue and can increase metabolic rate and heat production.[52] This suggests that our white adipose tissue can become metabolically trained and more metabolically active.

Mood

E xercise can also make a significant impact on mood, sleep restoration, and energy. Depression is a common psychiatric disorder. The World Health Organization estimates that more than 350 million people in the world are affected by depression. Finding tools to treat this illness can have a positive global impact. The case in the beginning of the chapter is an example of how exercise can elevate neurotransmitters (signal messengers) and good energy hormones called endorphins.

Endorphins are opioid-like chemicals in the body that can attach to cell receptors and release natural painkillers or analgesics but can also elevate mood. Studies have shown that endorphins are released when we feel pain and experience stress, such as exercise.[53] Studies using positron emission tomography (PET scans) have shown specific binding of opioid-like substances in specific areas of the brain following strenuous exercise.[54] (Exercise, then, can give you a high without the harm!) A PET scan is a diagnostic test that utilizes a radioactive tracer that hooks onto a biologically active molecule, such as a white cell or glucose molecule. It can see the function of tissues instead of just the anatomy.

We release endorphins in direct proportion to our level of exertion, and they act on our brains to create a sense of euphoria. This mechanism is thought to be the reason for a runner's high, which is based on a reward mechanism for prolonged exercise. Endorphins also inhibit the pain response; therefore, the pain of prolonged exercise is often not apparent until after exercise is finished. Endorphins also raise our pain thresholds, which allows us to perform in times of pain.

Neurotransmitters, such as serotonin, dopamine, and norepinephrine, are associated with mood disorders. Many medications used for treating depression target these transmitters. A major review examined 39 different studies to determine the role of exercise in depression. They found that exercise is moderately more effective for reducing symptoms of depression than no therapy at all.[55] Other organizations, such as the Association of Medicine and Psychiatry, have recommended that primary care doctors strongly advocate exercise to help reduce symptoms in their depressed patients.[56]

One public health study showed jogging in groups may be effective in improving the outlook of adolescent females with depressive symptoms.[57] The benefits from the natural elevation of neurotransmitters, such as mood stabilization and sleep promotion, may eliminate the need for medications in some cases. Exercise provides a potent mood stabilizer without the side effects seen with many medications, such as weight gain and sexual dysfunction.

Cognition

One of the most exciting benefits of aerobic exercise is its role in the elevation of brain-derived neurotrophic factor (BDNF). It is located in the brain and spinal cord and supports the growth and survival of neurons or nerve cells. The protein helps these cells grow and mature and increases efficiency of the connection between neurons. Research shows that BDNF is vital to neuroplasticity, which is the way in which the brain adapts to new challenges in learning and forming memory. Interestingly, BDNF is found in areas of the brain that control eating, drinking, and body weight. It's likely that it plays a role in the management of these issues as well. Aerobic exercise has been shown to elevate BDNF levels and improve neuroplasticity.[58]

Studies have also attributed elevations in BDNF to increases in the volume of different parts of the brain, such as the hippocampus (a part of our brain that deals with memory) and gray and white matter in the cortex (in charge of higher functions). In a time when more than 30 percent of Medicare beneficiaries report cognitive impairment or severe dementia, tools like exercise can be very valuable in the prevention of cognitive decline.[59] There are no guarantees, but research shows promise that a regular exercise regimen may help prevent age-related loss of brain volume and support cognitive health.[60]

Novel Ways to Exercise

We often hear, "I don't have time to exercise. Who has an hour to go to the gym?" It is true that an ounce of prevention is worth a pound of treatment—we want to remind readers that even a little goes a long way. In studies, bouts of moderate to intense exercise in 10-minute intervals up to 30 minutes a day can still bestow health benefits, especially when someone is first starting to exercise after living a sedentary lifestyle.[61,62,63] Another novel way to train more efficiently is high-intensity interval training. This is a modality that uses repeated episodes of high intensity from five seconds to eight minutes, followed by varying recovery periods. You can try this interval training with any endurance activity, such as biking, running, and cycling. It has been shown to reduce body fat percentages and reduce blood pressure and resting heart rates.[64,65] It causes reductions in biomarkers, such as cholesterol and glucose, as well as lowering inflammatory markers of IL-6 and TNF levels.[66] Researchers believe this benefit is realized when exercise intensity is varied, but the total energy expenditure of the workout increases.

Tabata is a popular method of high-intensity interval training (HIIT), which utilizes 20 seconds of high-intensity exercise alternated with 10 seconds of rest. One workout set (or Tabata) is a repetition of this cycle eight times for a total of four minutes. The number of Tabatas can be increased to last anywhere from 20 to 60 minutes based on your fitness level. It allows our bodies to work out at higher heart rates, which is better for our heart, and fitness levels. At the same time, it lowers the potential for injury because those high rates are balanced by lower intensity rates. More importantly, no adverse effects have been reported. This workout also typically lowers high-impact risk to joints and produces fewer injuries, since the time spent in high-intensity workouts is less.[67] This technique is also available through several Tabata apps you can use to devise your own HIIT workout.

Stretching and Balance

Stretching and balance work also are integral forms of exercise. Stretching induces flexibility, the ability to move a joint through its complete range of motion. Working on flexibility allows for utilizing the working function of a muscle as long as possible because you'll be able to move it farther for longer periods of time. With muscles, we must use them or lose them; we need to reinforce them to maintain their strength.

Balance helps prevent falls and injuries during other activities. It is likely the most undervalued and underutilized component of fitness. As we age, our bodies lose muscle mass, and the nerves in our extremities become less sensitive. The capabilities of the vestibular system in the inner ear also diminish. The vestibular system coordinates information from our senses and nerves, and tells our brain about motion and spatial orientation, and aids with balance. These age-related changes increase our predisposition to falling.

Exercises such as tai chi and qigong (types of meditative movement), along with yoga, have been shown to improve physical function, flexibility, and balance.[68] They often impact positively on quality of life for those with chronic disease, improve pain and movement in people with osteoarthritis, and help to remedy fatigue and depression.

THE BENEFIT OF ADDING A FOOD PLAN TO EXERCISE

Combining dietary changes and exercise can be integral to weight loss because doing both together can reduce the percentage of fat in the body and build muscle mass. This in turn improves metabolic rate. In addition, having an optimal food plan along with an exercise program can be critical for maintaining weight loss over time.

Exercise and Bone Loss

One major illness that affects more people than cardiovascular disease and cancer is osteoporosis or thinning of the bones, which creates a high risk of fragility fracture. Fifty percent of women in menopause will get osteoporosis. Twenty percent of those diagnosed with osteoporosis are men. A hip fracture is more dangerous than it seems.

It results in a very high mortality rate due to inactivity, loss of function, infection risk, and potential clot formation in the immobile limb. It is critical that we have tools to prevent bone loss and do weight-bearing exercises, such as weight lifting, walking, running, and yoga. High-impact exercises can build bone while low-impact exercises can keep bones strong as well.[69] Strengthening exercises, such as weight work and yoga, can develop muscle strength and balance, which is important for preventing falls.

Cancer Prevention

Regular physical exercise has been scientifically proven to help prevent certain cancers. Extensive studies have been conducted regarding breast and colorectal cancers, showing that the more we exercise, the lower our cancer risk.[70] In addition, we know there is a relationship between exercise and a reduction in endometrial, prostate, and lung cancers. Even with a cancer diagnosis, exercise has shown to help increase survival rates by 50 to 60 percent, again with the greatest impact on breast and colorectal cancers.[71]

In a study of prostate cancer patients, adding exercise to chemotherapy regimens was found to offset consequences of therapies that inhibit testosterone to decrease tumor size. These chemotherapy regimens block testosterone and decrease testosterone's ability to grow prostate cancer. Suppressing testosterone, however, can result in lower muscle mass, decreased functional performance, and decreased cardiorespiratory fitness. However, researchers showed that when exercise was added to therapies for prostate cancer patients, their cancer did not grow and the side effects of medication were also avoided.[72]

GET A GREEN THUMB

Gardening is a physical activity that boosts our heart rates and has a workload of about 4.5 to six METs. The *American Journal of Public Health* studied the health benefits of community gardening and saw that it helped people maintain a healthy body weight.[73] Many gardeners also find great satisfaction in this activity, and it aids their mental health. If you can find an activity you love, such as gardening, you probably will do it more often.

Play

A dults tend to forget the role of free play because we are so focused on productive tasks and being responsible. Playing in the yard with pets or kids, making a snowman, pillow fighting, running in the yard, and blowing bubbles are all examples of activities that raise your heart rate. Even a very enthusiastic game of charades can be both a physical activity and mentally stimulating as well. If you can find a physical activity that you also enjoy, you can easily make it a regular part of your life.

Along with joyful play, the role of laughter also has been studied. We know how good laughter can make us feel. Studies have shown that laughter can give us joy by raising our pain threshold, elevating our endorphins, and improving our mood, but it also exercises the diaphragm, which is a muscle.[74] Surprisingly, working your diaphragm by simply laughing can be a form of exercise!

How Do I Start Exercising?

Y ou may say, "That's great; there are a lot of benefits to exercise, but how do I start an exercise regimen when I feel so tired all the time?" This is a common question we hear frequently. It can be overwhelming to think of moving 150 minutes a week, as many experts recommend. The goal is to start with 10 minutes. Take a new, longer route from the parking lot to work. Stand and do slow movements during TV commercials, and do Kegel exercises (pelvic floor crunches) while sitting in your chair at work. Play catch with your kids or grandkids, or start dancing to music. You can start doing diaphragmatic breathing several times per day.

It is sometimes easier to initiate a new habit when we feel accountable. Try wearing an activity tracker. A variety of products on the market count your steps, evaluate the quality of your sleep, measure calories burned and floors climbed, and record the intensity of your activity. You can choose a device that matches your needs.

You can always start with a simple, inexpensive pedometer and monitor your steps. The goal for most people is 10,000 steps per day. You will be shocked at how few steps you take in a day, especially if you have a desk job. People who tell us they walk all the time usually

FIGURE 9   10 Recommended Exercises for Alignment/Posture

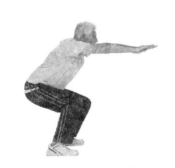

Exercise usually becomes a segue to other healthier habits

1 SEATED CHEST STRETCH

Body weight exercise that primarily targets your thighs (quadriceps, hamstrings), buttocks (gluteal muscles), and calves

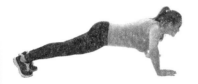

2 PUSH-UPS

Body Weight exercise that targets your upper body and core (abdominal/back) muscles.

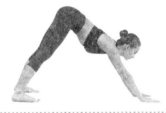

3 DOWNWARD DOG

Stretching and strengthening yoga pose—energizes the body—calms the brain and helps relieve stress.

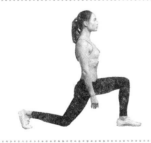

4 FRONT LUNGE

Focuses on strengthening of the lower body, balance, coordination, and flexibility.

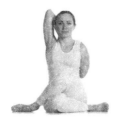

5 SEATED CHEST STRETCH

Improves posture, reduces tight muscles in the chest, and helps to strengthen upper body muscles to reduce kyphosis.

| FIGURE 9 | 10 Recommended Exercises for Alignment/Posture |

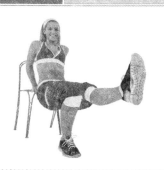

6 SEATED HIP MARCH

Strengthens hips and thigh muscles by sitting on the edge of chair and alternate lifting one leg (bent knee) off the floor as high as possible.

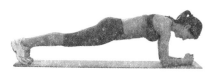

8 BODY PLANK

A floor exercise that works your whole body as you fight against gravity, primarily focusing on your core muscles.

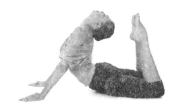

7 PRONE COBRA

Lie on your stomach and engage your core as you lift arms out to side and legs up simultaneously.

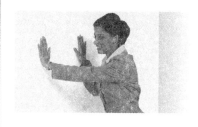

9 DOOR FRAME STRETCH

Similar to seated chest stretch, but for this one you're standing. Stretches out chest, shoulders, and back.

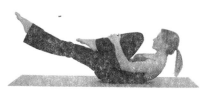

10 STRAIGHT LEG RAISE

Lie on your back, lift 1 or 2 legs together will determine the flexibility of hamstrings which can affect posture and alignment and if low back pain is present.

clock between 2,000 to 3,000 steps per day. You also will be surprised when you see how easy it is to increase your steps by going for a walk at lunchtime, parking farther away from the door, or taking the stairs instead of riding the elevator.

We have found our patients really respond to knowing their step counts every day because it gives them goals. Get creative. Make exercise social—something fun, an activity you look forward to. Small steps along a new path will take you to a new, fun destination. At the same time, you must learn to walk before you run. Start slowly and build each week. For those who do not walk much, start by walking to the corner of your block several times a day. Then add walking around the block and work toward a goal of 30-minute intervals five times per week. You can do this.

YOUR PRESCRIPTION

DEVELOPING YOUR OWN EXERCISE PROGRAM

1. Start with low intensity and go slow.

2. Change it up, and continue to challenge yourself. Change your workout and intensity as you get stronger.

3. A complete workout is more than just getting your heart rate up. Add resistance and strengthen your core. Sometimes balance training has health benefits that are as important as aerobics. Recovery is very important too.

4. Learn to laugh and play!

CHAPTER

15

The Benefits of Fasting

How fasting can help reset the immune system

The increasing abundance of our food supply over the last several centuries has contributed to excesses of eating. We have shifted away from eating at mealtimes and moved toward eating throughout the day—and for some, through the night. We see more obesity, and with that obesity there are increased risks for cardiovascular disease, cancer, and other chronic illnesses.

These days people typically eat three meals a day, along with periods of snacking and grazing in between. With that, our calorie consumption has become very high. When we eat, our food breaks down to glucose for our bodies to use as energy. The glucose our bodies don't utilize for energy is converted into fat. The common solution to being overweight is to consider how to reduce body fat: to either increase the expenditure of calories through exercise or to reduce calorie intake. Time-restricted fasting is an option to reduce the amount of time when calories are consumed even when there may not be a large reduction in the number of calories consumed.[1]

Fasting is an age-old concept that is defined as abstaining from certain foods or drinks for a period of time. Historically, fasting was used in religious observances and has been mentioned in sacred texts such as the Bible, Torah, and Quran. People have also used fasting as a form of nonviolent protest, such as when Mahatma Gandhi fought for India's independence.

In nature, animals commonly fast. Rodents, for instance, eat their food over several hours, then fast for about 20 hours per day.[2] Predatory animals will gorge after a large kill, then go for several days without eating again. Animals may also fast during times of illness or injury, only taking in nourishment when their healing crisis is over.

When we eat, food breaks down into glucose (sugars) and our body uses this as energy. This is considered a low ketone state. Glucose that is not used is turned to fat as triglycerides. On the other hand, during fasting, there is no glucose that the body can use for essential tasks, so the body uses triglycerides and breaks them down into free fatty acids and glycerol. The body uses these free fatty acids as energy. This is considered a high ketone state. Ketones can affect growth factors and molecules that are known to affect aging. For example, they can stimulate a growth factor that appears to have a role in long-term memory, Alzheimer's, psychiatric illness, and potentially with aging.[2]

There are several different types of fasting. *Intermittent fasting* is an umbrella term referring to periods lasting 12 to 48 hours with no caloric intake alternating with periods of regular eating. Intermittent fasting is different from *periodic fasting*, where there is no caloric intake for 2 to

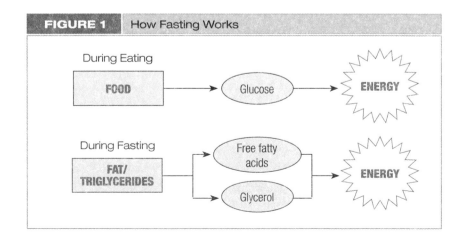

FIGURE 1   How Fasting Works

During Eating

FOOD → Glucose → ENERGY

During Fasting

FAT/TRIGLYCERIDES → Free fatty acids / Glycerol → ENERGY

FIGURE 2	Different Types of Fasting	
INTERMITTENT	**PERIODIC**	**TIME RESTRICTED FEEDS**
Alternate Day Fasts—alternate water only days with regular intake	2 to 21 days	12 hour fast—eat for 12 hour windows
5:2—take 500-600 calories two days per week alternating with regular intake	Water fasts— clinically monitored by physicians	16:8—eat during an 8 hour window

21 days. Common examples of intermittent fasting are caloric intake reduced to 500 to 600 calories two days per week and normal intake for five days. Alternatively, it can be zero caloric intake for two 24-hour cycles over a seven-day period and normal eating on the other days. *Time-restricted feeding* involves eating for short periods of time every day. For example, you might only eat during a 6- to 12-hour period during the daytime and fast the other 12 to 18 hours.

We are big fans of intermittent fasting and time-restricted feeding. Dr. R often does intermittent fasting, and Dr. A practices time-restricted feeding; both of us recommend these methods to our patients. Even if overall caloric intake doesn't decrease with time-restricted feeding, studies show there is still improvement in glucose regulation (blood sugar levels), blood pressure, heart rates, endurance, and loss of abdominal fat. This benefit appears to come from the change in metabolism that occurs when someone goes from a period of eating to a period of fasting.[3]

Multiple studies have looked at how fasting improves the health of rodents, larger animals, and even humans (although there are only a few studies on humans to date). They've shown reductions in body weight,[4,5] total cholesterol,[6,7] triglycerides,[7,8] and glucose,[6,9] with time-restricted feeding. In rats, reductions in inflammatory markers were also seen.[10]

What is even more interesting is that during fasting there appears to be repair of DNA and the removal of damaged or unwanted particles (autophagy), as well as an increased level of antioxidant protection and a reduction of inflammation. Both the process of autophagy and the action of antioxidants are key for fighting free radicals, oxidants, and cancer cells![11] In rats, fasting cycles increased the diversity of their gut bacteria, which are thought to be protective against obesity and other metabolic diseases.[12]

Fasting also has a role in increasing endurance. In some small animals, fasting was also shown to improve balance and coordination. In a trial of men, one group did resistance training and no fasting, one group did just time-restricted feeding for eight hours, and one group did both. The study showed that after thirty days, the men who did both lost both fat mass and weight. Interestingly, the resistance training only and the fasting group only showed no differences.[13] In a study of older adults with mild cognitive impairment, a fasting regimen helped improve verbal memory over time![14]

In addition, working out while fasting also improves the amount of fat burning during periods of exercise and appears to reduce appetite following workouts. In essence, fasting can increase the weight loss benefits of exercise.[15,16]

Summary and Benefits

1. Improved insulin sensitivity (reduced risk of diabetes)

2. Weight loss, reduction of fat, and reduction of abdominal circumference

3. Improved blood pressure

4. Improved cholesterol levels

5. Reduction of oxidative stress and inflammation

6. Increased removal of cellular debris (autophagy)

7. Improved endurance

8. Improved memory

YOUR PRESCRIPTION

1. Start with a 12-hour fast—no food from 7:00 p.m. to 7:00 a.m. Every four weeks, increase the fasting period by one to two hours.

2. Please consult with your doctor before you start fasting, especially if you have diabetes and are on insulin, so he or she can assess your medical condition and help you adjust your medications, if necessary.

3. Incorporate workouts while fasting if your physician approves.

4. Only drink water or tea during fasting; this will help curb your appetite.

Most people are pleasantly surprised at how easy this 12-hour window is. Often, after a few weeks, they are able to decrease the window for eating to eight hours per day. Don't worry if getting to eight hours is too difficult; do the best you can. There are so many potential benefits to fasting, so give it a try and see if you like the way you feel and change.

16

Optimism

"A pessimist sees the difficulty in every opportunity; an optimist sees the opportunity in every difficulty."

WINSTON CHURCHILL

Many of us consider challenges to be obstacles that keep us from the things we want. Those of us who are optimists tend to see the opportunity in those obstacles. In other words, an optimist will always believe that there is something positive to be gained regardless of the situation. An optimist will look for and find alternate solutions to problems, which can be satisfying and quite empowering.

If we take this statement to heart, we can see that optimism has many deeper applications than simply creating a good mood. Imagine how this positive outlook could help change how we view our own health. As discussed in earlier chapters, stress is a part of life, but what if we could use optimism as an added tool to deal with stress? What if by simply changing how we approach the stressors in our lives we could affect the toll stress takes on our bodies?

As we try to find tools for ourselves and our patients, optimism is a tool that is powerful, yet so often underutilized. Many people are optimistic when things are going well, such as when they have good health. But they find being optimistic difficult when their health is poor. Many think optimism is genetic, that you are born with a fixed outlook. You either have it or you don't. People often say, "Well, this is just how I was born" or "I can't change how I feel." But research shows that although there is a genetic component, optimism can also be cultivated, grown, and expanded.[1]

Can Optimism Improve Health?

A meta-analysis of 83 studies showed optimism, as well as reduced rates of depression and heart disease, were associated with improved health outcomes in cancer and pregnancy.[1,2,3] Optimists are found to be more resilient to stress, and newer research suggests a link between optimism and increased lifespan![4,5]

A potential reason for these improvements is that optimists make better lifestyle choices—they eat better and exercise more, they have more coping strategies to get through times of hardship, and they have more problem-solving capability to overcome adversity. All this information compels us to find ways to increase our optimism and make it another valuable tool for health! Let's look deeper at this.

How Do We Become Optimists?

You may be thinking, "Well, this is all well and good. But wanting to have positive emotions and social connectedness is one thing. Actually, having them is totally another." So how do we work on these positive thoughts? How do we improve optimism? In his book *Learned Optimism*, Martin Seligman, PhD, a pioneer in the field of positive psychology, gives many pointers to help us become more optimistic. He discusses practical exercises to decrease negative self-talk and challenges the way we view negative thoughts and beliefs. He teaches us to cultivate gratitude and positive emotions by actively shifting our minds from looking at the negative to finding the positive in any situation.

CONSIDER 1

✓ Self-talk is that voice in our head that is always criticizing us. Can we learn to make that voice go away?

How do we build lasting benefits from these concepts? Most of us make lists at the start of a new year to make changes, but we soon revert back to our old habits. Tal Ben-Shahar, a Harvard researcher, author, and professor who teaches leadership, happiness, and mindfulness all around the world, stated in an interview for NBC's *Today*, "Research shows that to bring about lasting change what we need [. . .] are the three R's—reminders, repetition, and rituals." Setting a reminder on your phone to turn your focus to the change you want to incorporate and doing these things on a regular basis lead to the changes in our brains. It trains our brains to create rituals that then allow us to keep up with the habits without much effort.

One of his students, Shawn Achor, outlined these tools to help achieve these changes in his book *The Happiness Advantage*, and in his TED Talk, "The Happiness Advantage."

1. **Keep a gratitude journal.** Every night, without the television on or any music or conversation in the background, write down three things that made you feel grateful and gave you joy. This can be small, such as a warm blanket, wonderful-tasting coffee, or a great nap. Refrain from using negative or positive comments like "I didn't do that badly today." Make sure to spend a moment reliving the reason it brought you joy.

2. **Exercise.** If you don't routinely exercise, try to move for at least five minutes every day. Set a clock and walk every day. If you can't walk, maybe jump around a pool or sit in a chair and move your arms and legs. Do that for two weeks. Then increase to eight minutes or more as you can. Exercise elevates dopamine, which improves our optimism.[6] There are more suggestions in chapter 17.

3. **Meditate.** Meditation definitely reduces our stress hormone, cortisol, and increases positive emotions. People are a little afraid of this one because they imagine that they have to be sitting in a lotus pose, with eyes closed, and go into a supernatural state. This is absolutely not the case! Please see page 142 on meditation, and try some of those exercises.

4. **Practice random acts of kindness.** Send an email or letter to thank someone you may not have fully thanked. Surprise someone with lunch or

a coffee, compliment someone you notice seems happy, or just give a smile as you walk by. Just because.

Reinforcing Positive Psychology

The World Health Organization defines health as not the absence of illness but a state of physical, mental, and social well-being. There is much research being done in the field of positive psychology. Positive psychology focuses on identifying the parts of life that make us want to keep living and functioning optimally, which in turn leads to well-being. It is the stuff that makes us happy to be alive. Martin Seligman categorizes positive psychology and well-being into five measurable pillars.[7] In his work, he challenges us to go beyond our basic desire to not get sick and instead work toward being well. He teaches us to focus on fulfillment, which raises the bar and makes us grow. Optimism and positive emotions are the link between positive psychology and physical health and ultimately our well-being.

There are five pillars of positive psychology:

- **Positive emotions.** Positive emotions are those which include a deeper feeling of emotion and purpose, such as gratitude, serenity, hope, awe, interest, pride, and amusement. Think of yourself and how you feel when you look at a beautiful natural landscape. What are the emotions you feel? These emotions are associated with the feel-good communicators in our bodies, known as dopamine and serotonin.[8]

- **Engagement.** Engagement is the complete immersion into an activity or job that can challenge us and our skills. It is the state where we lose ourselves in tasks.

- **Meaning.** Belong to and serve something that has a purpose larger than ourselves, a purpose for a greater good, such as community work.

- **Relationships.** Cultivate strong relationships with family, friends, and community.

- **Accomplishments.** Work toward mastery and success for the sake of achievement.

Just as a building cannot be held up with only one or two pillars, neither are only one or two of these pillars enough for us to get the most out of life. A building needs a proper foundation, and so do we. A proper foundation for us is all five pillars of positive psychology. For example, for a pleasant or fulfilled life, one must cultivate social connections, work toward goals that are in line with passions, and find meaning on a day-to-day level. An optimistic outlook is a great aide in achieving these pillars.

Triggering Our Fire

There is also a link between negative emotions, such as depression, and increased inflammatory markers.[9,10] The negative emotions of depression and anxiety can also elevate cortisol, our stress hormone.[11] In essence, negative emotions can refuel the internal fire we discussed in earlier chapters that continues to signal more inflammation in our bodies by contributing to sympathetic overdrive. Although this seems like common sense, it is one more reason to work toward reducing our negative emotions by working on increasing our positive ones like optimism.

Cultivating these practices can rewire the way your brain thinks about a situation.[8] On any given day, there are situations that are out of our control that may induce stress. As Michael Singer says in his book *The Surrender Experiment*, "Each of us actually believes that things should be the way we want them, instead of being the natural result of all the forces of creation."

Ultimately, the only things in our control are our thoughts, which lead to our emotions. The practices on page 191 can lead to a more positive outlook. A more positive outlook can help us achieve the foundation of the five pillars. By focusing on what we can control—doing work with intent, having gratitude for what we do have and where we are, and allowing the natural course of things to go forward—we will find that we are more peaceful and fulfilled. The tools can be a challenge for anyone, regardless of whether you are a naturally positive person or not. We know there is a limited time in the day. We know we cannot sit and meditate and exercise all day. As the late Richard Edlich, MD, a former plastic surgeon at the University of Virginia and Dr. A's mentor, once told her, "It is not about finding the calm [and joy] on a mountain in India. That's easy. It is about bringing the calm into the here and now." Working on rituals teaches us how to bring calm into our daily lives. Like anything worth doing, with time and practice these tasks will begin to feel natural, and you will be astonished at your changes. Give it a try!

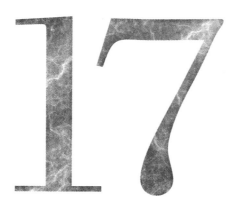

Recharge

Eat well, play more, sleep deeply, heal

A healthy body is a body in balance: the balance between eustress and distress, the balance between the sympathetic fight-or-flight and parasympathetic rest-and-recharge systems, and the balance between resource depletion and replenishment. We must maintain that balance to be healthy—to achieve homeostasis.

While stress is a normal part of life, most of us have created lives for ourselves in which we are constantly on the go. We are overstimulated by electronics and work. We multitask. We handle large amounts of emotional stress. We eat poorly. We don't sleep enough. We deprive our bodies of that balance, and this leads to inflammation and ultimately illness.

Learning how to maintain balance is a true art. Taking time to recharge the body with rest, yoga, meditation, and exercise is essential. Eating nourishing foods, slowing down our pace, and learning the beauty of taking our time are vital steps to counterbalancing all these depletive sources of stress in our lives. We live in a world where stress is worn as a badge of honor. We are proud of how well we perform on little sleep and how little we need to manage. We are proud of our go, go, go and play hard mentalities. Ultimately, however, the balance is shifted and we get sick. It is inevitable. It happened to Dr. A and so many others, and it will happen to you—unless you change. Change is hard. For so many people, taking the time to rest and recharge is looked at as a sign of weakness.

We argue that that mentality has to change. We chose to take back our lives, and we wear our rest-and-recharge time as our badges of honor—because without that balance, the body cannot heal.

The process will be slow, but each day, take one step. Try to find 20 minutes to deep breathe. Try to put your electronics away 15 minutes before bed. Try to go for a walk. Try to eliminate processed foods and meats, to start. Even with small steps, you will start to feel different—better. Small steps will lead to big steps.

With this book, we give you the tools you need to live your life well, with energy and without illness. This is what we want for you. With the best in mind for you, be well. Nourish your body, your microbiome, and your soul. Rest. Take time to play and sleep. Eat abundantly and well.

Best,
Monica and Jyothi

CHAPTER 4

1. Selye H. Stress and the general adaptation syndrome. *Br Med J*. 1950;1(4667): 1383–1392.

2. Schneiderman N, Ironson G, Siegel SD. Stress and Health: Psychological, behavioral, and biological determinants. *Annu Rev Clin Psychol*; 2005; 1: 607–628.

3. Donoho CJ, Weigensberg MJ, Emken BA. Stress and abdominal fat: preliminary evidence of moderation by the cortisol awakening response in Hispanic peripubertal girls. *Obesity*; May 2011; 19(5): 946–952.

4. Schbacher K, O'Donovan A, Wolkowitz O et al. Good stress, bad stress and oxidative stress: insights from anticipatory cortisol reactivity. *Psychoneuroendocrinology*; Sept 2013; 38(9): 1698–708.

5. Miller GE, Cohen S, Ritchey AK. Chronic psychological stress and the regulation of pro-inflammatory cytokines: a glucocorticoid–resistance model. *Health Psychol*; Nov. 2002; 21 (6):531–41.

6. Harbuz MS, Chover-Gonzalez AJ, Jessop DS. Hypothalamo-pituitary–adrenal axis and chronic immune activation. Ann. NY *Acad Sci* 2003; 992: 99–106.

7. Epel E, Blackburn EH, Lin J, Dhabhar FS, Adler NE et al. Accelerated telomere shortening in response to life stress. *PNAS*; December 2004; 101 (49): 17312–315.

CHAPTER 5

1. Top 10 causes of death fact sheet. World Health Organization 5/2014; http://www.who.int/mediacentre/factsheets/fs310/en/

2. Flegal KM, Carroll MD, Kit BK, Ogden CL. Prevalence of obesity and trends in the distribution of body mass index among US adults, 1999–2010. *JAMA*; 2012; 307(5):491–97.

3. https://www.cdc.gov/media/releases/2017/p0718-diabetes-report.html

4. Clinical Guidelines on the Identification, Evaluation, and Treatment of Overweight and Obesity in Adults. *The Evidence Report*. NIH publications. No. 98–4083. September 1998.

5. Vogel R, Corretti M, Plotnick GD. Effect of a single high-fat meal on endothelial function in healthy subjects. *American Journal of Cardiology*; February 1997; 79 (3): 350–354.

6. Shah B, Ganguzza L, Slater J et al. The Effect of a Vegan versus AHA DiEt in Coronary Artery Disease (EVADE CAD) trial: study design and rationale. *Contemp Clin Trials Commun*. 2017 Dec;8:90–98.

7. Estruch R, Ros E, Salas-Salvadó J et al. Primary Prevention of Cardiovascular Disease with a Mediterranean Diet. *N Engl J Med* 2013; 368:1279–1290.

8. Enos WF, Holmes RH, Beyer J. Coronary disease among United States soldiers killed in action in Korea: preliminary report. *JAMA*; 1953; 152: 1090–1093.

9. McNamara JJ, Molot MA, Stremple JF, Cutting RT. Coronary artery disease in combat casualties in Vietnam. *JAMA*; 1971; 216: 1185–1187.

10. Calle E, Rodriguez C, Walker-Thurmond K, Thun MJ. Overweight, obesity, and mortality from cancer in a prospectively studied cohort of U.S. adults. *N Engl J Med*; 2003; 348:1625–1638.

11. Gallup-Healthways Well-Being Index, 2009.

12. Flegal K, Kit B, Orpana H, Graubard B. Association of all-cause mortality with overweight and obesity using standard body mass index: A systematic review and meta-analysis. *JAMA*; Jan 2013. Jan 2;309(1):71–82.

13. Prospective Studies Collaboration. Body-mass index and cause-specific mortality in 900,000 adults: collaborative analyses of 57 prospective studies. *Lancet*. 2009; Mar 28; 373(9669):1083–96.

14. Goldstein DJ, Beneficial health effects of modest weight loss, *Int J Obes Relat Metab Disord*. June 1992: 397–415.

15. CDC. Vital signs: prevalence, treatment, and control of high levels of low-density lipoprotein cholesterol. United States, 1999–2002 and 2005–2008. *MMWR*; 2011; 60(4):109–14.

16. Whelton P, Carey R, Aronow W et al. 2017 ACC/AHA/AAPA/ABC/ACPM/AGS/APhA/ASH/ASPC/NMA/PCNA Guideline for the Prevention, Detection, Evaluation, and Management of High Blood Pressure in Adults: A Report of the American College of Cardiology/American Heart Association Task Force on Clinical Practice Guidelines. *J Am Coll Cardiol* 2018;71:e127-e248.

17. Hubert HB, Feinleib M, McNamara PM, Castelli WP. Obesity as an independent risk factor for cardiovascular disease: a 26-year follow-up of participants in the Framingham Heart Study. *Circulation*; 1983; 67: 968–97.

18. Danner FW. A national longitudinal study of the association between hours of TV viewing and the trajectory of BMI growth among US children. *J Pediatr Psychol*; 2008; 33: 1100-7.

CHAPTER 6

1. Robinson CJ, Bohannan BJM et al. From structure to function: the ecology of host-associated microbial communities. *Microbiology and Molecular Biology Reviews*; 9/2010; 74(3): 453–6.

2. Cho I, Blaser MJ. The Human Microbiome: at the interface of health and disease. *Nat Rev Genet*. 2012; 13(4): 260–270.

3. V Hooper LV, Gordon JI. Commensal host-bacterial relationships in the gut. *Science*; 292:1115–1118

4. Ursell LK, Metcalf JL, Parfrey LW, Knight R. Defining the human microbiome. *Nutrition Reviews*. 2012 Aug 1;70(suppl_1):S38–44.

5. Ou J, Carbonero F, Zoetendal EG et al. Diet, microbiota, and microbial metabolites in colon cancer risk in rural Africans and African Americans. *American Journal of Clinical Nutrition*. 2013 Jul 1;98(1):111–20.

6. O'Keefe SJ, Li JV, Lahti L et al. Fat, fibre and cancer risk in African Americans and rural Africans. *Nature Communications*. 2015 Apr 28;6:6342.

7. Tang WH, Wang Zeneng et al., Intestinal Microbial Metabolism of Phosphatidylcholine and Cardiovascular Risk. *NEJM*; 2013; 368: 1575–84.

8. Berk M, Williams LJ, Jacka FN et al. So depression is an inflammatory disease, but where does the inflammation come from? *BMC Medicine*; 2013; 11:200, 1–16.

9. Pussinen PJ, Havulinna AS, Lehto M et al. Endotoxemia is associated with an increased risk of incident diabetes. *Diabetes Care*; 2011;34(2):392–397.

10. Naito E, Yoshida Y, Makino K   et al., Beneficial effect of oral administration of lactobacillus casei strain shirota on insulin resistance in diet-induced obesity mice. *Journal of Applied Microbiology*; 2011;110(3):650–657.

11. Zhang R et al., *J Neuroimmunol*; 2009; (206): 121–4.

12. Emanuele E et al., *Neuroscience Letters*; 2010; 471: 162–5.

13. Vaarala O, Leaking gut in type 1 diabetes. *Curr Opin Gastroenterol*; 2008; 24(6): 701–6.

14. Cani PD, Bibiloni R, Knauf C et al. Changes in gut microbiota control metabolic endotoxemia-induced inflammation in high-fat diet-induced obesity and diabetes in mice. *Diabetes*; 2008;57(6):1470–1481.

15. Vaziri ND. CKD impairs barrier function and alters microbial flora of the intestine: a major link to inflammation and uremic toxicity. *Curr Opin Nephrol Hypertens*; 2012 Nov;21(6):587–92.

16. Stilling RM, Dinan TG, Cryan JF. Microbial genes, brain and behavior-epigenetic regulation of the gut-brain axis. *Genes, Brain and Behavior*; 2014; 13:69–86.

17. Critchfield JW, van Hemert S, Ash M, Mulder L, Ashwood P. The Potential Role of Probiotics in the Management of Childhood Autism Spectrum Disorders. *Gastroenterology Research and Practice*. 2011, Volume 201, Article ID 161358.

18. Strachan DP. Hay fever, hygiene, and household size. *BMJ*; 1989; 299: 1259–1260.

19. Blaser MJ Who are we? Indigenous microbes and the ecology of human diseases. *EMBO 2006*, Rep 7:956–960.

20. Salminen S, Gibson C, Bouley MC et al., Gastrointestinal physiology and function: the role of prebiotics and probiotics. *Br J Nutr*; 1998; 80(Suppl 1):S147–71.

21. Savaiano DA, Abou EA, Smith DE, Levitt MD. Lactose malabsorption from yogurt, sweet acidophilus milk, and cultured milk in lactose deficient individuals. *Am J Clin Nutr*; 1984; 40:1219–23.

22. Goldin BR, Gorbach SR. Clinical indications for probiotics: an overview. Clinical Infectious Diseases; 2008; 46:S96–100.

23. Guandalini S, Pensabene L, Zikri MA et al., Lactobacillus GG administered in oral rehydration solution to children with acute diarrhea: a multicenter European trial. *J Pediatr Gastroenterol Nutr*; 2000; 30:54–60.

24. Hilton E, Kolakowski P, Singer C, Smith M. Efficacy of lactobacillus GG as a diarrheal preventive in travelers. *J Travel Med*; 1997; 4:41–3.

25. Kalliomaki M, Salminen S, Arvilommi H et al. Probiotics in primary prevention of atopic disease: a randomized placebo-controlled trial. Lancet; 2001; 357:1076–9.

26. Goldin BR, Gorbach SR. Clinical indications for probiotics: an overview. *Clinical Infectious Diseases*; 2008; 46:S96–100.

27. Hatakka K, Martio J, Korpela M et al., Effects of probiotic therapy on the activity and activation of mild rheumatoid arthritis—a pilot study. *Scand J Rheumatol*; 2003; 32:211–5.

28. Mandel DR, Eickas K et al., Bacillus coagulans: a viable adjunct therapy for relieving symptoms of rheumatoid arthritis according to a randomized, controlled trial. *BMC Complement Altern Med*; 2010; 10: 1.

29. Liu Y, Tran DQ, Rhoads JM. Probiotics in disease prevention and treatment. *Journal of Clinical Pharmacology*. 2018 Oct;58:S164–79.

CHAPTER 7

1. Wilson Tang WH, Wang Z, Levison BS et al. Intestinal Microbial Metabolism of Phosphatidylcholine and Cardiovascular Risk. *N Engl J Med* 2013; 368: 1575–1584.

2. Pan A, Sun Q, Bernstein AM et al. Red meat consumption and mortality results from 2 prospective cohort studies. *Arch Intern Med*, 2012;172(7):555–563.

3. Kleinbongard P, Dejam A, Lauer T et al. Plasma nitrite concentrations reflect the degree of endothelial dysfunction in humans. *Free Radic Biol Med*. 2006; 40(2): 295–302.

4. Pereira EC, Ferderbar S, Bertolami MC et al. Biomarkers of oxidative stress and endothelial dysfunction in glucose intolerance and diabetes mellitus. *Clin Biochem*. 2008; 41(18): 1454–1460.

5. Esselstyn CB, Gendy G, Doyle J et al. A way to reverse CAD? *Journal of Family Practice*. July 2014; 63(7): p356–36b.

6. Skog K, Steineck G, Augustsson K, Jägerstad M. Effect of cooking temperature on the formation of heterocyclic amines in fried meat products and pan residues. *Carcinogenesis*, 1995; 16(4): 861–867.

7. Cross AJ, Pollock JR, Bingham SA. Haem, not protein or inorganic iron, is responsible for endogenous intestinal N-nitrosation arising from red meat. *Cancer Res*. 2003; 63(10): 2358–2360.

8. Kromhout D, Bosschieter EB, Coulander CdL. The inverse relation between fish consumption and 20-year mortality from coronary heart disease. *N Engl J Med*, 1985; 312: 1205–1209.

9. Marckmann P, Gronbaek M. Fish consumption and coronary heart disease mortality: a systematic review of prospective cohort studies. *Eur J Clin Nutr*. 1999; 53: 585–90.

10. Cerqueira MT, Fry MM, Connor WE. The food and nutrient intakes of the Tarahumara Indians of Mexico. *Am J Clin Nutr*, 1979; 32: 905–915.

11. Campbell T. *The China Study*. BenBella Books, Inc; 2006.

12. Deopurkar R, Ghanim H, Friedman J et al. Differential effects of cream, glucose, and orange juice on inflammation, endotoxin, and the expression of Toll-like receptor-4 and suppressor of cytokine signaling-3. *Diabetes Care*, May 2010; 33(5): 991–7.

13. Song M, Fung TT, Hu FB et al. Association of animal and plant protein intake with all-cause and cause-specific mortality. *JAMA Internal Medicine*. 2016 Oct 1;176(10):1453–63.

14. Michaëlsson K, Wolk A, Langenskiöld S et al. Milk intake and risk of mortality and fractures in women and men: cohort studies. *BMJ*; 2014; 349: g6015.

15. Sonestedt E, Wirfalt E, Wallstrom P et al. Dairy products and its association with incidence of cardiovascular disease: the Malmo diet and cancer cohort. *Eur J Epidemiol*; 2011; 26: 609–18.

16. Huth PJ, Park KM. Influence of dairy product and milk fat consumption on cardiovascular disease risk: a review of the evidence. *Adv Nutr*; 2012; 3: 266–85.

17. Feskanich D, Willett WC, Stamper MJ, Colditz GA. Milk, dietary calcium, and bone fractures in women: a 12-year prospective study. *Am J Pub Health*; June 1997, 87 (6): 992–7.

18. Bischoff-Ferrari HA, Baron, JA, Burckhardt P et al. Calcium intake and hip fracture risk in men and women: a meta-analysis of prospective cohort studies and randomized control trials. *Am J Clin Nutr*, 2007; 86(6): 1780–90.

19. Weaver, C, Plawecki, K. Dietary calcium adequacy of a vegetarian diet. *American Journal of Clinical Nutrition*; 1994; 1238S–41S.

20. Feskanich D, Willett WC, Stamper MJ, Colditz GA. Protein consumption and bone fractures in women. *Am J Epidemiol*. 1996; 143: 472–79.

21. Dietary guidelines at http://www.health.gov/dietaryguidelines/dga2005/document/html/appendixB.htm

22. Heaney RP, Weaver CM. Calcium absorption from kale. *AJCN*; 1990; 51: 656–7.

23. Calcium and milk: what's best for your bones and health? *Nutrition Source*, Harvard School of Public Health.

24. Feskanich D, Weber P, Willett WC et al. Vitamin K intake and hip fractures in women: a prospective study. *Am J Clin Nutr*. 1999; 69: 74–79.

25. Booth SL, Tucker KL et al. Dietary vitamin K intakes are associated with hip fracture but not with bone mineral density in elderly men and women. *Am J Cl Nutr*. 2000; 71: 1201–08.

26. Hannan MT, Tucker KL, Dawson-Hughes B et al. Effect of dietary protein on bone loss in elderly men and women: the Framingham Osteoporosis Study. *J Bone Miner Res*. 2000 Dec;15(12):2504–12.

27. Lampe JW. Dairy products and cancer. *J Am Coll Nutr*. 2011; 30(5 Suppl 1): 464S–70S.

28. Genkinger JM, Hunter DJ, Spiegelman D et al. Dairy products and ovarian cancer: a pooled analysis of 12 cohort studies. *Cancer Epidemiol Biomarkers Prev.* 2006; 15: 364–72.

29. Giovannucci E, Rimm EB. Calcium and fructose intake in relation to risk of prostate cancer. *Cancer Res*; 1998; 58: 442–447.

30. Giovannucci E, Liu Y, Platz EA et al. Risk factors for prostate cancer incidence and progression in the Health Professionals Follow-up Study. *International Journal of Cancer*; 2007; 121: 1571–78.

31. Danby FW. Nutrition and Acne. *Clinics in Dermatology*; November–December 2010; 28 (6): 598–604.

32. Campbell, T. *The China Study.* BenBella Books, Inc. 2006, p. 60–61.

33. Michaëlsson K, Wolk A, Langenskiöld S et al. Milk intake and risk of mortality and fractures in women and men: cohort studies. *BMJ*; 2014; 349: g6015.

34. Kumar M, Kumar A, Nagpal R et al. Cancer-preventing attributes of probiotics: an update. *Int J Food Sci Nutr*; 2010; 61: 473–96.

35. US Department of Commerce, US Census Bureau, *The 2012 Statistical Abstract*, report number 217 found at http://www.census.gov/compendia/statab/cats/health_nutrition/food_consumption_and_nutrition.html

36. American Heart Association, found at http://www.heart.org/HEARTORG/GettingHealthy/NutritionCenter/HealthyDietGoals/Sugars-and-Carbohydrates_UCM_303296_Article.jsp

37. University of Texas, SALSA study, found at http://www.uthscsa.edu/hscnews/singleformat2.asp?newID=3861

38. University of Texas, SALSA study, found at http://www.uthscsa.edu/hscnews/singleformat2.asp?newID=3861

39. Swithers S. Artificial sweeteners produce the counterintuitive effect of inducing metabolic derangements. *Trends in Endocrinology and Metabolism*, September 2013; 24 (9): 431–441.

40. Suez J, Korem T, Zeevi D et al. Artificial sweeteners induce glucose intolerance by altering the gut microbiota. *Nature*; October 2015, 514: 181–186.

41. Aris, A & Leblanc S. Maternal and fetal exposure to pesticides associated to genetically modified foods in Eastern Townships of Quebec. *Reprod Toxicol*. 2011 May; 31(4): 528–33.

42. Centers for Disease Control and Prevention (CDC). Investigation of human health effects associated with potential exposure to genetically modified corn. A report to the US Food and Drug Administration from the Centers for Disease Control and Prevention. *National Center for Environmental Health*; 2001.

43. Ornish D, Scherwitz LW et al. Intensive lifestyle changes for reversal of coronary heart disease. *JAMA.* 1998 Dec 16;280(23):2001–7.

CHAPTER 8

1. Lee JH, Khor TO et al. Dietary Phytonutrients and Cancer Prevention: NRF2 signaling, epigenetics and cell death mechanisms in blocking cancer imitation and progression. *Pharmacol Ther*, Feb 2013; 137 (2): 153–171.

2. Giovannucci E, Rimm EB et al. A prospective study of tomato products, lycopene and prostate cancer risk. *J Natl Cancer Inst*; 2002 Mar; 694(5): 391–8.

3. Karppi J, Laukkanen JA et al. Serum lycopene decreases the risk of stroke in men. *Neurology*, 2012 Oct; 79(15): 1540–47.

4. Johnson EJ. The role of carotenoids in human health. *Nutr Clin Care*, 2002; Mar-April; 5(2):56–65.

5. Hertog MG, Feskens EJ et al. Dietary antioxidants flavonoids and risk of coronary heart disease: the Zutphen Elderly Study. *Lancet*. 1993; 342: 1007–1011.

6. Knekt P, Jarvinen R et al. Flavonoid intake and coronary mortality in Finland: a cohort study. *BMJ*, 1996; 312: 478–81.

7. Semba RD, Ferrucci L. et al. Resveratrol levels and all-cause mortality in older community-dwelling adults. *JAMA Intern Med*. 2014 July; (174(7): 1077–84.

8. World Health Organization. Diet, nutrition, and the prevention of chronic diseases. Geneva: World Health Organization, 1990.

9. Joshipura KJ, Hu FB, Manson JE et al. The effect of fruit and vegetable intake on risk for coronary heart disease. *Ann Intern Med*. 2001; 134: 1106–14.

10. Leenders M, Sluijs I, Ros MM et al. Fruit and vegetable consumption and mortality: European prospective investigation into cancer and nutrition. *Am J Epidemiol*. 2013; 178: 590–602.

11. Oyebode O, Gordon-Dseagu V et al. Fruit and vegetable consumption and all cause, cancer and CVD mortality: analysis of Health Survey for England data. *J Epidemiol Community Health*; 2014 Sep;68(9):856–62.

12. Dauchet L, Amouyel P, Hercberg S et al. Fruit and vegetable consumption and risk of coronary heart disease: a meta-analysis of cohort studies. *J Nutr*, 2006; 136: 2588–93.

13. Hu FB, Stampfer MJ et al. Dietary intake of alpha-linolenic acid and risk of ischemic heart disease among women. *Am J Clin Nutr*, 1999; 69: 890–7.

14. Liu S, Burin JE et al. A prospective study of dietary fiber intake and risk of cardiovascular disease among women. *JACC 2002*; 39: 49–56.

15. Liu S, Stampfer MJ et al. Whole grain consumption and risk of coronary heart disease: results from the Nurses' Health Study. *Am J Clin Nutr*, 1999; 70: 412–419.

16. Berni Canini R, Di Costanzo M et al. Potential beneficial effects of butyrate in intestinal and extraintestinal diseases. *World J Gastroenterol*, Mar 28, 2011; 17(12): 1519–1528.

17. Ledikwe JH, Blanck HM, Kettel Khan L et al. Dietary energy density is associated with energy intake and weight status in US adults. *Am J Clin Nutr*, 2006; 83: 1362–8.

18. Research to Practice Series No 5, Low-energy-dense foods and weight management: cutting calories while controlling hunger. National Center for Disease Control Prevention and Healthy Promotion.

19. Duncan KH, Bacon JA, Weinsier RL. The effects of high and low energy density diets on satiety, energy intake, and eating time of obese and nonobese subjects. *American Journal of Clinical Nutrition*, 1983; 37: 763–767.

20. Shintani TT, Beckham S, Brown AC, O'Connor HK. The Hawaii Diet: ad libitum high carbohydrate, low fat multi-cultural diet for the reduction of chronic disease risk factors: obesity, hypertension, hypercholesterolemia, and hyperglycemia. *Hawaii Medical Journal*, 2001; 60: 69–73.

21. Ornish D, Scherwitz LW et al. Intensive lifestyle changes for reversal of coronary heart disease. *JAMA*, December 16, 1998—Vol 280, No. 23.

22. Kushi LH, Lenart EB et al. Health implications of Mediterranean diets in light of contemporary knowledge. 1. Plant foods and dairy products. *Am J Clin Nutr*, June 1995, 61: 1407S–1415S.

23. Hu FB, Willett WC. Optimal diets for prevention of coronary heart disease. *JAMA*; 2002 Nov 27; 288(20): 2569–78.

24. de Lorgeril M, Renaud S, Mamelle N et al., Mediterranean alpha-linolenic acid-rich diet in secondary prevention of coronary heart disease. *Lancet*, 1994; 343: 1454–9.

25. Appel L, Moore TJ, Obarzanek E, for the DASH Collaborative Research Group. A clinical trial of the effects of dietary patterns on blood pressure. *N Engl J Med*, 1997; 336: 1117–24.

26. Jacobs DR Jr, Meyer KA, Kushi LH, Folsom AR. Whole-grain intake may reduce the risk of ischemic heart disease death in postmenopausal women: the Iowa Women's Health Study. *Am J Clin Nutr*, 1998; 68: 248–57.

27. Liu S, Stampfer MJ, Hu FB et al. Whole-grain consumption and risk of coronary heart disease: results from the Nurses' Health Study. *Am J Clin Nutr*, 1999; 70: 412–9.

28. Fung TT, Willett WC, Stampfer MJ et al. Dietary patterns and risk of coronary heart disease in women. *Arch Intern Med* 2001; 161: 1857–62.

29. Hu FB, Rimm EB, Stampfer MJ et al. Prospective study of major dietary patterns and risk of coronary heart disease in men. *Am J Clin Nutr*, 2000; 72: 912–21.

30. Crous-Bou M, Fung TT, Prescott J et al. Mediterranean diet and telomere length in Nurses' Health Study: population based cohort study, *BMJ*, Dec 2014, 349.

31. Mann, T, Tomiyama J, Westling E et al. *American Psychologist*, Vol 62(3), Apr 2007; 220–233.

32. Joshi S, Ostfeld RJ, McMacken M. The Ketogenic Diet for Obesity and Diabetes—Enthusiasm Outpaces Evidence. *JAMA Intern Med.* 2019;179(9): 1163–1164.

33. National Institute of Diabetes and Digestive and Kidney Disease, Weight Control Information Network, found at http://win.niddk.nih.gov/publications/myths.htm

CHAPTER 9

1. Anitschkov NN. A history of experimentation on arterial atherosclerosis in animals. In: Blumenthal HT ed. *Cowdry's Arteriosclerosis: A Survey of the Problem*. 2nd ed. Springfield Ill: Charles C Thomas; 1967: 21–44.

2. McGill HC. The relationship of dietary cholesterol to serum cholesterol concentration and to atherosclerosis in man. *Am J Clin Nutr*, 1979; 32: 2664–2702.

3. Hu FB, Willett WC. Optimal diets for prevention of coronary heart disease. *JAMA*; 2002 Nov 27; 288(20): 2569–78.

4. Gordon T: The diet-heart idea: outline of a history. *Am J Epidemiol*, 1988; 127: 220–225.

5. Hu FB, Stampfer MJ, Manson JE et al. Dietary saturated fats and their food sources in relation to the risk of coronary heart disease in women. *American Journal of Clinical Nutrition*. 1999 Dec 1;70(6):1001–8.

6. Tang WW, Wang Z, Levison BS et al. Intestinal microbial metabolism of phosphatidylcholine and cardiovascular risk. *New England Journal of Medicine*. 2013 Apr 25;368(17):1575–84.

7. Arnett DK, Blumenthal RS, Albert MA et al. 2019 ACC/AHA guideline on the primary prevention of cardiovascular disease: a report of the American College of Cardiology/American Heart Association Task Force on Clinical Practice Guidelines. *Journal of the American College of Cardiology*. 2019 Sep 2;74(10):e177-232.

8. Dehghan M, Mente A, Zhang X et al. Associations of fats and carbohydrate intake with cardiovascular disease and mortality in 18 countries from five continents (PURE): a prospective cohort study. *Lancet*. 2017 Nov 4;390(10107): 2050–62.

9. Gianos E, Williams KA, Freeman AM, Kris-Etherton P, Aggarwal M. How pure is PURE? Dietary lessons learned and not learned from the PURE Trials. *American Journal of Medicine*. 2018 May 1;131(5):457–8.

10. Satija A, Bhupathiraju SN, Spiegelman D et al. Healthful and unhealthful plant-based diets and the risk of coronary heart disease in US adults. *Journal of the American College of Cardiology*. 2017 Jul 17;70(4):411–22.

11. Sacks FM, Lichtenstein AH, Wu JH et al. Dietary fats and cardiovascular disease: a presidential advisory from the American Heart Association. *Circulation*. 2017 Jul 18;136(3):e1–23.

12. Bhatt DL, Steg PG, Miller M et al. Cardiovascular risk reduction with icosapent ethyl for hypertriglyceridemia. *New England Journal of Medicine*. 2019 Jan 3;380(1):11–22.

13. Kang JX, Leaf A. Antiarrhythmic effects of polyunsaturated fatty acids: recent studies. *Circulation*,1996; 94: 1774–1780.

14. Connor SL, Connor WE. Are fish oils beneficial in the prevention and treatment of coronary artery disease? *Am J Clin Nutr*, 1997; 66(4 suppl): 1020S–1031S.

15. Kromhout D, Bosschieter EB, de Lezenne Coulander C. The inverse relation between fish consumption and 20-year mortality from coronary heart disease. *N Engl J Med*,1985; 312: 1205–1209.

16. Pietinen P, Ascherio A, Korhonen P. et al. Intake of fatty acids and risk of coronary heart disease in a cohort of Finnish men: the ATBC Study. *Am J Epidemiol*, 1997; 145: 876–887.

17. Ascherio A, Rimm EB, Giovannucci EL et al. Dietary fat and risk of coronary heart disease in men: cohort follow-up study in the United States. *BMJ*, 1996; 313: 84–90.

18. Steinberg D, Parthasarathy S, Carew TE et al. Beyond cholesterol: modifi-cations of low-density lipoprotein that increase its atherogenicity. *N Engl J Med*, 1989; 320: 915–924.

19. Mozaffarian D, Rimm EB, Herrington DM. Dietary fats, carbohydrate, and progression of coronary atherosclerosis in postmenopausal women. *Am J Clin Nutr*, 2004; 80: 1175–1184.

20. Mensink RP, Katan MB. Effect of dietary fatty acids on serum lipids and lipo-proteins: a meta-analysis of 27 trials. *Arterioscler Thromb*, 1992; 12: 911–919.

21. Harris WS, Mozaffarian D et al. Omega-6 fatty acids and risk for cardiovas-cular disease. *Circulation*, 2009; 119: 902–907.

22. Laaksonen DE, Nyyssonen K, Niskanen L et al. Prediction of cardiovascular mortality in middle-aged men by dietary and serum linoleic and polyunsatu-rated fatty acids. *Arch Intern Med*. 2005; 165: 193–199.

23. Harris WS, Mozaffarian D et al. Omega-6 fatty acids and risk for cardiovas-cular disease. *Circulation*, 2009; 119: 902–907.

24. Simopoulos AP. An Increase in the Omega-6/Omega-3 Fatty Acid Ratio In-creases the Risk for Obesity. *Nutrients*. 2016;8(3):128.

25. Mensink RP, Katan MB. Effect of dietary trans fatty acids on high-density and low-density lipoprotein cholesterols levels in healthy subjects. *NEJM*, 1990; 323: 439–445.

26. Nestel P, Noakes M et al. Plasma lipoprotein and Lp [a] changes with substitu-tion of elaidic acid for oleic acid in the diet. *J Lipi Res*, 1992; 33: 1029–1036.

27. Katan MB, Zock PL. Trans fatty acids and their effects on lipoproteins in humans. *Annu Rev Nutr*,1995; 15: 473–493.

28. Salmeron J, Hu FB, Manson JE et al. Dietary fat intake and risk of type 2 diabetes in women. *Am J Clin Nutr*, 2001; 73: 1019–1026.

29. Kushi LH, Lew RA, Stare FJ. et al. Diet and 20-year mortality from coronary heart disease: the Ireland-Boston Diet-Heart Study, *N Engl J Med*,1985; 312: 811–818.

30. Hu FB, Stampfer MJ, Manson JE et al. Dietary fat intake and the risk of cor-onary heart disease in women. *N Engl J Med*, 1997; 337: 1491–1499.

31. Estruch R, Ros E et al. Primary prevention of cardiovascular disease with a Mediterranean diet. *NEJM*, April 2013; 368: 14; 1279–90.

32. Kris-Etherton PM for the Nutrition Committee. *Circulation*;1999;100: 1253–58.

33. Rudel L, Parks J et al. Compared with dietary monounsaturated and satu-rated fat, polyunsaturated fat protects African green monkeys from coronary artery atherosclerosis. *Arteriosclerosis, Thrombosis, and Vascular Biology*, 1995; 15: 2101-2110.

34. Novick J. https://www.pritikin.com/your-health/healthy-living/eating-right/1103-whats-wrong-with-olive-oil.html#.VF5MF_J0yP8

35. Vogel R, Coretti M et al. The postprandial effect of components of the Medi-terranean diet on endothelial function. *J Am Coll Card*, 2000; 36: 1455.

36. Trichopoulou A, Barnia C et al. Anatomy of health effects of Mediterranean diet: Greek EPIC prospective cohort study. *BMJ*, 2009; 338: b2337.

37. Assunção ML, Ferreira HS et al. Effects of dietary coconut oil on the biochemical and anthropometric profiles of women presenting abdominal obesity. *Lipids*. 2009 Jul;44(7):593-601.

38. Ros E, Nunez I et al. A walnut diet improves endothelial function in hypercholesterolemic subjects. *Circulation*, 2004; 109: 1609–1614.

39. Fraser G, Sabate J et al. A possible protective effect of nut consumption on risk of coronary heart disease: The Adventist Health Study. *Arch Intern Med*, 1992; 152(7): 1416–1424.37. Assunção ML, Ferreira HS et al. Effects of dietary coconut oil on the biochemical and anthropometric profiles of women presenting abdominal obesity. *Lipids*, Jul; 44(7): 593–601.

40. Sabate J, Fraser GE et al. Effects of walnuts on serum lipid levels and blood pressure in normal med. *NEJM*, 3/1993; 328(9): 603–7.

41. Hu F, Stampfer M et al. Frequent nut consumption and risk of coronary heart disease in women: prospective cohort study. *BMJ*, 1998; 317: 1341.

42. Sabate J, Oda K et al. Nut consumption and blood lipid levels: A Pooled Analysis of 25 Intervention Trials. *Arch Intern Med*, 2010; 170(9): 821–82.

43. Ros E, Nunez I et al. A walnut diet improves endothelial function in hypercholesterolemic subjects. *Circulation*, 2004; 109: 1609–1614.

44. Alpher CM, Mattes RD. Peanut consumption improves indices of cardiovascular disease risk in healthy adults. *J Am Clin Nutr*, 22: 2; 2003.

45. Jenkins D, Kendall C et al. Dose response of almonds on coronary heart disease risk factors: blood lipids, oxidized low-density lipoproteins, lipoprotein(a), homocysteine, and pulmonary nitric oxide. *Circulation*. 2002; 106: 1327–1332.

46. Zatónski W, Campos H, Willett W. Rapid declines in coronary heart disease mortality in Eastern Europe are associated with increased consumption of oils rich in alpha-linolenic acid. *Eur J Epidemiol*, 2008; 23: 3–10.

47. Campos H, Baylin A, Willett WC. Alpha-linolenic acid and risk of nonfatal acute myocardial infarction. *Circulation*, 2008; 118: 339–345.

CHAPTER 10

1. Sanchez E, Kelley KM. *Herb and Spice History*. Penn State College of Agricultural Sciences, Department of Horticulture, http://extension.psu.edu/plants/gardening/fact-sheets/herbs/herb-and-spice-history/extension_publication_file

2. Kuptniratsaikul V, Dajpratham P et al. Efficacy and safety of curcuma domestica extracts compared with ibuprofen in patients with knee osteoarthritis: a multicenter study. *Clin Interv Aging*, 2014; 9: 451–8.

3. Hu Wang, Tin Oo Khor et al. Plants Against Cancer: A Review on Natural Phytochemicals in Preventing and Treating Cancers and Their Druggability. *Anticancer Agents Med Chem*. 2012 Dec; 12(10): 1281–1305.

4. Fratiglioni L, De Ronchi D, Agüero-Torres H. Worldwide prevalence and incidence of dementia. *Drugs Aging*, 1999 Nov; 15(5):365–75.

5. Yang F, Lim GP, Begum AN et al. Curcumin inhibits formation of amyloid beta oligomers and fibrils, binds plaques, and reduces amyloid in vivo. *J Biol Chem*. 2005 Feb 18; 280(7):5892–901.

6. Hewlings, S, Kalman, D. Cucurmin: A review of its' effects on human health. *Foods*. 2017 Oct; 6(10): 92.

7. Min Y, Kwang HH, et al. Curcumin attenuates adhesion molecules and matrix metalloproteinase expression in hypercholesterolemic rabbits. *Nutrition Research*, Volume 34, Issue 10, October 2014; pp 886–893.

8. Puangsombat K, Smith JS. Inhibition of heterocyclic amine formation in beef patties by ethanolic extracts of rosemary. *J Food Sci.*, 2010 Mar;75(2): T40–7.

9. Khan A, Safdar M et al. Cinnamon improves glucose and lipids of people with type 2 diabetes. 10.2337/diacare.26.12.3215 *Diabetes Care*, December 2003; vol. 26 no. 12 3215–3218.

10. Couturier K, Batandier C. Cinnamon improves insulin sensitivity and alters the body composition in an animal model of the metabolic syndrome. *Arch Biochem Biophys*, 2010 Sep 1; 501(1): 158–61.

11. Cheng SS, Liu JY et al. Chemical polymorphism and antifungal activity of essential oils from leaves of different provenances of indigenous cinnamon. *Bioresour Technol*, January 2006: pp 306–312.

12. Rosti L, Gastaldi G, Frigiola A. Cinnamon and bacterial enteric infections. *Ind J Ped*, 2008, 75: 529–530.

13. Zhu M, Carvalho R, Scher A, Wu CD. Short-term germ-killing effect of sugar-sweetened cinnamon chewing gum on salivary anaerobes associated with halitosis. *J Clin Dent*, 2011, 22: 23–26.

14. Jayaprakasha GK, Jagan Mohan Rao L, Sakariah KK. Volatile constituents from cinnamomum zeylanicum fruit stalks and their antioxidant activities. *J Agric Food Chem* 2003; 51: 4344–4348.

15. Rahman K, Lowe GM. Garlic and cardiovascular disease: a critical review. *J Nutr*, March 2006;136(3):736S–740S.

16. Stevinson C, Pittler MH, Ernst E. Garlic for treating hypercholesterolemia. a metaanalysis of randomised clinical trials. *Ann Intern Med*, 2000;19: 420–9.

17. Breithaupt-Grogler K, Ling M, Boudoulas H et al. Protective effect of chronic garlic intake on elastic properties of aorta in the elderly. *Circulation*, 1997; 96: 2649–55.

CHAPTER 11

1. Askew EW, University of Utah, healthcare.utah.edu/publicaffairs/news

CHAPTER 12

1. Sleep at the Wheel: The Prevalence and Impact of Drowsy Driving. *AAA Foundation for Traffic Safety*, November 2010, https://aaafoundation.org/wpcontent/uploads/2018/02/2010DrowsyDrivingReport.pdf

2. Hirshkowitz M, Whiton K, Albert S M, et al. National Sleep Foundation's sleep time duration recommendations: methodology and results summary. *Sleep Health*. 2015 Mar;1(1):40–43.

3. Spiegel K, Leproult R, Van Cauter E. Impact of sleep debt on metabolic and endocrine function. *Lancet*. 1999; 354: 1435–1439.

4. Sleep foundation. www.sleepfoundation.org

5. Vgontzas AN, Zoumakis E et al. Adverse effects of modest sleep restriction on sleepiness, performance, and inflammatory cytokines. *J CLin Endocrinol Metab.* 2004; 89(5): 2119.

6. Tsai K, Hsu TG, Lu FJ et al. Age–related changes in the mitochondrial depolarization induced by oxidative injury in human peripheral blood leukocytes. *Free Radic Res*, 2001; 35: 251–255.

7. Teixeira, K.R.C., dos Santos, C.P et al. Night workers have lower levels of antioxidant defenses and higher levels of oxidative stress damage when compared to day workers. *Sci Rep 9*, 4455 (2019).

8. Everson C, Laatsch CD, Neil H. Antioxidant defense responses to sleep loss and sleep recovery. *Am J Phsiol Regul Integr Comp Physiol*, 2005; 288: R374–383.

9. Liebler DC, Reed DJ. Free-radical defense and repair mechanisms. *Free Radical Toxicology*, edited by Wallace KB. Washington, DC: Taylor & Francis. 1997; p141–171.

10. Everson CA, Laatsch CD, Hogg N. Antioxidant defense responses to sleep loss and recovery. *American Journal of Physiology*, 2005;288 (2):R374–383.

11. Droge W, Breitkreutz R. Glutathione and immune function. *Proc Nutr Soc.*, Nov 2000; 59(4): 595–600.

12. Summala H, Mikkota T. Fatal accidents among car and truck drivers: effects of fatigue. age, and alcohol consumption. From up to date definition and consequences of sleep deprivation, *Hum Factors.* 1994; 36(2): 315.

13. Van Dongen HP, Maislin G, Mullington JM, Dinges DF. The cumulative cost of additional wakefulness: dose–response effects on neurobehavioral functions and sleep physiology from chronic sleep restriction and total sleep deprivation. *Sleep*, 2003; 26(2): 117.

14. Jones M. How little sleep can you get away with? *New York Times Magazine*, April 15,2011.

15. Goel N, Rao H, Durmer JS, Dinges DF. Neurocognitive Consequences of Sleep Deprivation. *Semin Neurol*, 2009: 29(4):320–339.

16. Bonnet MH, Arand DL. We are chronically sleep deprived. *Sleep*, 1995; 18(10): 908.

17. Van Cauter E, Polonsky KS et al. Roles of circadian rhythmicity and sleep in human glucose regulation. *Endocr Rev.*,1997; 18(5): 716–738.

18. Taheri S, Lin L, Austin D, Young T, Mignot E. Short sleep duration is associated with reduced leptin, elevated ghrelin, and increased body mass index. *PLoS Med*, 2004; 1(3):e62

19. Scott EM, Carter AM, Grant PJ. Association between polymorphisms in the clock gene, obesity and the metabolic syndrome in man. *Int J Obes* (Lond), 2008; 32(4): 658–662.

20. Gangwisch J, Heymsfield S, Boden-Albala B et al. Sleep Duration as a Risk Factor for Diabetes Incidence in a Large US Sample. *Sleep*, 2007;30 (12): 1667–1673.

21. Knutson RL. Impact of sleep and sleep loss on glucose homeostasis and appetite regulation. *Sleep Med Clinic*. June 2007; 2(2):187–197.

22. Engle-Friedman M. The effects of sleep loss on capacity and effort. *Sleep Science* (2014), http://dx.doi.org/10.

23. Vgontzaz AN, Liao D. Pejovic S et al. Insomnia with short sleep duration and mortality: the Penn State cohort. *Sleep*, 2010; 33(9):1159.

24. Sleep disorders and sleep deprivation: an unmet public health problem, *Consensus Report*. March 2006. Biomedical and Health Research, Institute of Medicine of the National Academies.

25. Taheri S, Lin L, Austin D, Young T, Mignot E. Short sleep duration is associated with reduced leptin, elevated ghrelin, and increased body mass index. *PLoS Med*, 2004; 1(3):e62.

26. Nedeltcheva AV, Kilkus JM, Imperial J et al. Insufficient sleep undermines dietary efforts to reduce adiposity. *Annals of Internal Medicine*, 2010;153(7): 435–441.

27. Prince TM, Abel T. The Impact of Sleep Loss on Hippocampal Function. *Learning and Memory*. 2013, 20:558–569.

28. Gais S, Born J. Declarative memory consolidation: Mechanisms acting during human sleep, *Learning and Memory*, 2004, 11: 679–685.

29. Payne JD, Nadel L. Sleep, dreams, and memory consolidation: The role of the stress hormone cortisol. *Learn Mem*, Nov 2004; 11(6): 671-678.

30. Kumar R1, Birrer BV et al. Reduced mammillary body volume in patients with obstructive sleep apnea. *Neuroscience Lett*, 2008 June 27; 438(3): 330–334.

31. Kato M, Roberts-Thompson P, Philips BG, et al. Impairment of endothelium–dependent vasodilation of resistance vessels in patients with obstructive sleep apnea. *Circulation*, 200; 102: 2607–2610.

32. Srinivasan V, Pandi-Perumal SR, Brzezinski A et al. Melatonin Immune function and cancer. *Recent Pat Endocr Metab Immune Drug Discov*, 2011 May; 5(2):107–23.

33. Blask De. Melatonin, sleep disturbance and cancer risk. *Sleep Medicine Reviews*, 2009; 257–264.

34. Hansen J. Increased breast cancer risk among women who work predominantly at night. *Epidemiology*, 2001; (12): 74–77.

35. Feychting M, Osterlund B, Ahlbom A. Reduced cancer incidence among the blind. *Epidemiology*. 1998; (9): 490–494.

36. Chang AM, Aeschbach D, Duffy JF. Evening use of light-emitting eReaders negatively affects sleep, circadian timing, and next –morning alertness. *PNAS* 2015; 112 (4); 1232–1237.

37. Ackermann K, Bux R, Rub U et al. Melatonin synthesis in the human pineal gland. *BMC Neuroscience*. 2007 Mar,8 (1): P2.

38. Cajochen C, Munch M, Kobialka S et al. High sensitivity of human melatonin, alertness, thermoregulation and heart rate to short wavelength light. *J Clin Endo Met*,2005; 90: 1311–1316.

39. Figueiro MG, Bierman A, Plitnick B et al. Preliminary evidence that both blue and red light can induce alertness at night. *BMC Neuroscience*, 2009; 10: 105.

40. Dahl R E, Lewin D S. Pathways to adolescent health sleep regulation and behavior. *Journal of Adolescent Health*, 2002; 31 (6); 175–184.

41. Oakley, Barbara M. *A Mind for Numbers*. New York: Penguin Group. 2014. Print.

CHAPTER 13

1. Sengupta P. Health Impacts of Yoga and Pranayama: a state–of–the–art review. *Int J Prev Med*, Jul 2012; 3 (7): 444–458.

2. Ricard M, Lutz A, Davidson R. Mind of the meditator. *Scientific American*, 2014: 39-45.

3. Yogananda. *Autobiography of a Yogi*. Los Angeles, California: Self Realization Fellowship. 2006.

4. Gothe NP, Kramer AF, McAuley E. The effects of an 8 week Hatha yoga intervention on executive function in older adults. *J Gerontol A Biol Sci Med Sci*, 2014 Sep; 69(9): 1109–16.

5. Crow EM, Jeannot E, Trewhela A. Effectiveness of Iyengar yoga in treating spinal (back and neck) pain: a systematic review. *Int J Yoga*, 2015; 8(1): 3–14.

6. Banaski J, Williams H, Haberman M. Effect of Iyengar yoga practice on fatigue and diurnal salivary cortisol concentration in breast cancer survivors. *J Am Acad Nurse Pract*, 2011 Mar; 23(3): 135–42.

7. Yadav RK, Magan D, Mehta N. Efficacy of a short- term yoga-based lifestyle intervention in reducing stress and inflammation: preliminary results. *J Altern Complement Med*, 2012 Jul; 18(7): 662–667.

8. Thirthalli J, Naveen GH, Rao MG. Cortisol and antidepressant effects of yoga. *Indian J Psychiatry*, 2013 Jul; 55(3): S405–408.

9. Banasik J, Williams H, Haberman M et al. Effect of Iyengar yoga practice on fatigue and diurnal salivary cortisol concentration in breast cancer survivors. *J AM Acad Nurse Pract*, 2011 Mar; 23(3): 135–42.

10. Bhasin MK, Dusek JA, Chang E-H et al. Relaxation response induces temporal transcriptome changes in energy metabolism, insulin secretion and inflammatory pathways. *PLOS One*. 2013 May 1;8(5):e62817.

11. Creswell JD, Irwin MR, Burklund LJ. Mindfulness–based stress reduction training reduces loneliness and pro–inflammatory gene expression in older adults: a small randomized controlled trial. *Brain Behav Immun*, 2012 Oct; 26 (7): 1095–101.

12. Black DS, Cole SW, Irwin MR et al. Yogic meditation reverses NF-KB and IRF–related transcriptome dynamics in leukocytes of family dementia caregivers in a randomized controlled trial. *Psychoneuroendocrinology*, 2013 Mar; 38(3): 348–55.

13. Chatterjee S, Mondal S. Effect of regular yogic training on growth hormone and dehydroepiandrosterone sulfate as an endocrine marker of aging. *Evidence Based Complementary and Alternative Medicine*. 2014;2014:240581.

14. Sarvottam K, Magan D, Yadav RK et al. Adiponectin, interleukin-6 and cardiovascular disease risk factors are modified by a short–term yoga–based lifestyle intervention in overweight and obese men. *J Alter Complement Med*, 2013 May; 19(5): 397–402.

15. Nidhi R, Padmalatha V, Nagarathna R. Effect of a yoga program on glucose metabolism and blood lipid levels in adolescent girls with polycystic ovary syndrome. *Int J Gynaecol Obstet*, 2012 Jul; 118 (1): 37–41.

16. Sengupta, P. Health impacts of yoga and pranayama: a state-of-the-art review. *Int J Prev Med*, 2012 Jul; 3(7); 444–458.

17. Ghiadone L, Donald AE, Cropley M et al. Mental stress induces transient endothelial dysfunction in humans. Clinical Investigation and Reports. *Circulation*. 2000; 102: 2473–2478.

18. Sivasankara S, Pollard-Quintner S, Sachdeva PR et al. The effect of a six week program of yoga and meditation on brachial artery reactivity. Do psychosocial interventions affect tones. *Clin Clin Cardiol*, 2006; 29: 393–398.

19. Ornish D, Scherwitz LW, Doody RS. Effects of stress management training and dietary changes in treating ischemic heart disease. *JAMA*, 1983 Jan; 249(1): 54–59.

20. Cramer H, Lauche R, Haller H et al. A systematic review of yoga for heart disease. *European Journal of Preventive Cardiology*, 2015 Mar:22(3): 284–295.

21. Zernicke KA, Campbell TS, Blustein PK. Mindfulness–based stress reduction for the treatment of irritable bowel syndrome symptoms: a randomized waitlist controlled trial. *Int J Behav Med*, 2013 Sept; 20 (3) :385–96.

22. Goyal M, Singh S, Sibinga EMS. Meditation Programs for Psychological stress and Well-being. A Systematic Review and Meta-analysis. *JAMA*, 2014; 174 (3) : 357–468.

23. Jedel S, Hoffman A, Meriman P. A randomized controlled trial of mindfulness-based stress reduction to prevent flare-ups in patients with inactive ulcerative colitis. *Digestion*, 2014; 89(2): 142–55.

24. Lazar, SW, Kerr CE, Wasserman RU, et al. Meditation experience is associated with increased cortical thickness. *Neuroreport*, 2006 Nov; 16 (17): 1893–7.

25. Gottselig JM, Hofer-Tinguely G, Borbely AA, et al. Sleep and rest facilitate auditory learning. *Neurosci*, 2004; 127: 557–561.

26. Liu XC, Pan L, Hu Q et al. Effects of yoga training in patients with chronic obstructive pulmonary disease: a systematic review and metaanalysis. *J Thorac Dis*, 2014 Jun; 6(6): 795–802.

27. Berkowitz B, Clark P. The health hazards of sitting. *Washington Post*. Jan 2014.

28. Singh S, Kyizom T, Singh KP et al. Influence of pranayamas and yoga – asanas on serum insulin, blood glucose and lipid profile in type 2 diabetes. *Indian Journal of Clinical Biochemistry*, 2008; 22(4): 365–368.

29. Manjunatha S, Vempati RP, Ghosh D, Bijlani RL. An investigation into the acute and long–term effects of selected yogic postures on fasting and postprandial glycemia and insulinemia in healthy young subjects. *Indian J Physiol Pharmacol*, 2005; Jul-Sept: 49: (3): 319–24.

30. Singh, G, Singh J. Yoga Nidhra: a deep mental relaxation approach. *Br J Sports Med.* 2010; 44: i71–i72.

31. Walton KG., et al. Lowering cortisol and CVD risk in postmenopausal women: a pilot study using the Transcendental Meditation program. *Annals of New York Academy of Sciences.* 2005; 1032: 211–215.

32. Schneider RH. Altered responses of cortisol, GH, TSH and testosterone to acute stress after four months' practice of Transcendental Meditation. *Annals of the New York Academy of Sciences,* 1994; 746: 381–384.

33. Ray IB, Menezes AR, Malur AR, et al. Meditation and coronary heart disease: a review of the current clinical evidence. *The Ochsner Journal,* 2014; 14: 696–703.

34. Schneider RH, Grim CE, Rainforth MV et al. Stress reduction in the secondary prevention of cardiovascular disease: randomized controlled trial of Transcendental Meditation and health education in Blacks. *Circulation: Cardiovascular Quality and Outcomes,* 2012; 5: 750–758.

35. Brook, R D, Appel LJ, Rajagopalan S. Beyond medications and diet: alternative approaches to lowering blood pressure. A scientific statement from the AHA. *Hypertension.* 2013 Jun;61(6):1360–83.

36. Dangwal, Parmesh. *"I Dare!"*: *Kiran Bedi,*:Sangam, 2001. Print.

37. Brewington K. Yoga, meditation program helps city youth cope with stress. *The Baltimore Sun* Feb 2011: n. 2011. Print

38. Sullivan B, Thompson H. "Brain, Interrupted" *The New York Times.* 2013: n. page. Print

CHAPTER 14

1. Puetz TW. Physical activity and feelings of energy and fatigue: epidemiological evidence. *Sports Med,* 2006; 36(9): 767–80.

2. Conn VS, Hafdahl AR, Brown LM. Meta-analysis of quality of life outcomes from physical activity interventions. *Nurs Res,* 2009; 58(3): 175–83.

3. Garber CE, Blissmer B, Deschenes MR et al. Quantity and quality of exercise for developing and maintaining cardiorespiratory, musculoskeletal, and neuromotor fitness in apparently healthy adults: guidance for prescribing exercise. *Medicine & Science in Sports and Exercise,* 2011.

4. Haskell WL, Lee I-M, Pate RR et al. Physical activity and public health: updated recommendations for adults from the American College of Sports Medicine and the American Heart Association. *Circulation,* 2007; 116 (9):1081–1093.

5. General Physical Activities Defined by Level of Intensity. https://www.cdc.gov/nccdphp/dnpa/physical/pdf/PA_Intensity_table_2_1.pdf

6. Lee IM, Rexrode KM, Cook NR et al. Physical activity and coronary heart disease in women:is "no pain, no gain" passe? *JAMA* .2001; 285(11):1447–54.

7. Manson, JE, Greenland P, LaCroix AZ et al. Walking compared with vigorous exercise for the prevention of cardiovascular events in women. *N Engl J Med,* 2002; 347: 716–25.

8. Seeso HD, Paffenbarger RS Jr., Lee IM. Physical activity and coronary heart disease in men: the Harvard Alumni Health Study. *Circulation*, 2000; 102(9): 975–80.

9. Tanasescu M, Leitzmann MF, Rimm EB et al. Exercise type and intensity in relation to coronary heart disease in men. *JAMA*, 2002:288(16): 1994–2000.

10. US Department of Health and Human Services. 2008 Physical Activity Guidelines for Americans [Internet]. Washington (DC): ODPHP Publication No. UU0036.2008 [cited 2010 Oct 10]. 61p.

11. Healy GN, Dustan DQ, Salmon J et al. Breaks in Sedentary Time: Beneficial Associations with Metabolic Risk. *Diabetes Care*, April 2008; 31: 661–6.

12. Hales, C, Carroll, M, Fryar, C, Ogden, C. Prevalence of Obesity and Severe Obesity Among Adults: United States, 2017–2018, *NCHS Data Brief No. 360*, February 2020.

13. Warren TY, Barry V, Hooker SP et al. Sedentary behaviors increase risk of cardiovascular disease mortality in men. *Med Sci Sports Exerc*, 2010; 42(5): 879–85.

14. Teychenne M, Ball K, Salmon J. Sedentary behavior and depression among adults: a review. *Int J Behav Med*, 2010; 17(4): 246–54.

15. Healy GN, Dustan DQ, Salmon J et al. Television time and continuous metabolic risk in physically active adults. *Med Sci Sports Exerc*, 2008; 40 (4): 639–45.

16. US Department of Health and Human Services. Physical Activity Guidelines Advisory Committee Report, 2008[Internet]. Washington (DC): ODPHP Publication No. U0049. 2008[cited 2010 Sep 24]. 683p. Available from: http://www.health.gov/paguidelines/Report/pdf/CommitteeReport.pdf.

17. Whaley MH. *ACSM'S Guidelines for Exercise Testing and Prescription*, Seventh Edition. Baltimore, Maryland: Lippincott Williams & Wilkins, 2006.

18. Bravata DM, Smith-Spangler C, Sundaram V et al. Using pedometers to increase physical activity and improve health: a systematic review. *JAMA*,.2007; 298(19): 2296–304.

19. Kang M, Marshall SJ, Barreira TV, Lee JO. Effect of pedometer-based physical activity interventions: a meta–analysis. *Res Q Exerc Sport*, 2009: 80 (3): 648–55.

20. Owen N, Healy GN, Matthews CE, Dunstan QW, Too Much Sitting: Population- Health Science of Sedentary Behavior, *Exerc Sports Sci Rev*, July 2010; 35: 105–113.

21. https://www.mayoclinic.org/healthy-lifestyle/weight-loss/in-depth/exercise/art-20050999

22. Ainsworth BE, et al. 2011 compendium of physical activities: A second update of codes and MET values. *Medicine & Science in Sports & Exercise*. 2011;43:1575.

23. Boreham C. *The Physiology of Training*. UK: Elsevier Limited, 2006. Print.

24. Jenkins NT, Witkowski S, Spangenburg EE, Hagberg JM. Effects of acute and chronic endurance exercise on intracellular nitric oxide in putative endothelial progenitor cells: role of NAPDH oxidase. *Am J Physiol Heart Circ Physiol*, 2009 Nov; 297(5): 798–805.

25. McAllister RM, Newcomer SC, Laughlin H. Vascular nitric oxide: effects of exercise training in animals. *Applied Physiology, Nutrition, and Metabolism,* 2008; 33 (1): 173–178.

26. Jungersten L, Ambring A, Wall B, Wennmalm A. Both physical fitness and acute exercise regulate nitric oxide formation in healthy humans. *J Appl Physiol,* 1997; 82: 760–764.

27. De Franceschi MS, Palange AL, Mancuso A et al. Decreased platelet aggregation by shear stress stimulated endothelial cells in vitro: description of a method and first results in diabetes. *Diab Vasc Dis Res,* 2015 Jan;12(1):53–61.

28. Whyte G ed., *Physiology of Training.* Philadelphia: Churchill Livingston Elsevier, 2006.

29. Blomstrand E, Eliasson J, Karlsson HKR, Kohnke R. Branched-chain Amino Acids Activate Key Enzymes in Protein Synthesis after Physical Exercise. *J Nutr,* Jan 2006; 136: 269S–73S.

30. Sowers S. *A Primer on Branched Chain Amino Acids.* Huntington College of Health Sciences, 2009: 1-5.

31. Kreher JB, Schwartz JB. Overtraining Syndrome. *Sports Health,* Mar 2012; 4(2): 128-138.

32. Suleman A. "Exercise Physiology." emedicine.medscape.com. *Medscape.* Jul 2013.

33. Westby MD. A health professional's guide to exercise prescription for people with arthritis: a review of aerobic fitness activities. *Arthritis Care and Res,* 2001; 45(6): 501–511.

34. Hall J, Skevington SM, Maddison PJ et al. A randomized controlled trial of hydrotherapy in rheumatoid arthritis. *Arthritis Care Res,* 1996; 9(3): 206–215.

35. Bartels EM, Lund H, Hagen KB et al. Aquatic exercise for the treatment of knee and hip osteoarthritis. *Cochrane Database of Systematic Review.* 2007; 4: 1–9.

36. Pollock Ml, Franklin BA, Balady GJ et al. Resistance Exercise in Individuals With and Without Cardiovascular Disease. *Circulation,* 2000; 101: 828–833.

37. Ladkowsksi, Edward R. "Are Isometric Exercise a Good Way to Build Strength." Healthy Lifestyle Fitness, *Mayo Clinic,* 25 Nov 2014. Web. 9 Sept. 2014.

38. Menshikova EV, Ritov VB, Fairfull L et al. Effects of exercise on mitochondrial content and function in aging human skeletal muscle. *Gerontol A Biol Sci Med Sci,* June 2006; 61(6): 534–540.

39. Pool HA, Axford JS. The Effects of Exercise on the Hormonal and Immune Systems in Rheumatoid Arthritis, *Rheumatology,* 2001, 40: 610–614

40. Cumming DC, Brunsting LA, Strich G et al. Reproductive hormone increases in response to acute exercise in men. *Medicine and Science in Sports and Exercise,* 198618:369 -373.

41. Saugy M, Robinson N, Saudan C et al. Human growth hormone doping in sport, *Br J Sports Med.* July 2006; 40(Suppl 1): i35–i39.

42. Despres J-P. Obesity body fat distribution and risk of cardiovascular disease. *Circulation,* 2012; 125: 130–1313.

43. Klein S. The case of visceral fat–argument for the defense. *Journal of Clin Invest,* 2004; 113 (11): 1530–1532.

44. Whitworth JA, Williamson PA, Mangos G, Kelly JJ. Cardiovascular Consequences of Cortisol Excess. *Vasc Health Risk Manag*, Dec 2005; 1(4): 291–299.

45. Artinian NT, Fletcher GF, Mozaffarian D et al. Interventions to promote physical activity and dietary lifestyle changes for cardiovascular risk factor reduction in adults: a scientific statement from the American Heart Association. *Circulation*, 2010: 122: 406–441.

46. Ross R, Bradshaw AJ. The future of obesity reduction: beyond weight loss. *Nat Rev Endocrinology*, 2009: 5: 319–325.

47. Janiszewski PM, Ross R. Physical activity in the treatment of obesity: beyond weight reduction. *Appl Physiol Nutr Metab*, 2007; 32: 512–522.

48. Donoho CJ, Weigensberg MJ, Emken BA et al. Stress and abdominal fat: preliminary evidence of moderation by the cortisol awakening response in Hispanic peripubertal girls. *Obesity*, May 2011; 19(5): 946–952.

49. Donoho CJ, Weigensberg MJ, Emken BA et al. Stress and abdominal fat: preliminary evidence of moderation by the cortisol awakening response in Hispanic peripubertal girls. *Obesity*, May 2011; 19(5): 946–952.

50. Purnell JQ, Kahn SE, Samuels MH et al. Enhanced cortisol production rates, free cortisol, and 11B-HSD-1 expression correlate with visceral fat and insulin resistance in men: effect of weight loss. *Am J Physiol Endocrinol Metab*, Feb 2009; 296(2): E351–E357.

51. Stanford KI, Middelbeek RJW, Townsend KL et al. Brown adipose tissue regulates glucose homeostasis and insulin sensitivity. *J Clin Invest*, 2013; 123(1): 215–223.

52. Bostrom P, Wu J, Jedrychowski MP et al. A PGC1-alpha–dependent myokine that drives brown–fat- like development of white fat and thermogenesis. *Nature*, Jan 2012; 48(7382): 463–8.

53. Carr DB, Bullen BA, Skrinar GS et al. Physical condition facilitates the exercise–induced secretion of beta–endorphin and beta–lipotropin in women. *N Engl J Med*, 1981; 305: 560–563.

54. Boecker H, Sprenger T, Spilker ME et al. The runner's high: opioidergic mechanism in the human brain. *Cerebral Cortex*, 2008 Nov;18(11):2523–31.

55. Cooney GM, Dwan K, Greig CA et al. Exercise for depression. *Cochrane Database of Systematic Reviews*, 12 Sept 2013; Web. 10 Oct 2014.

56. Craft LL, Pernal FM. The benefits of exercise for the clinically depressed. The Primary Care Companion, *J Clin Psychiatry*, 2004; 6(3): 104–111.

57. Nabkasom C, Miyai N, Sootmongkol A, Junprasert S et al. Effects of physical exercise on depression, neuroendocrine stress hormones and physiological fitness in adolescent females with depressive symptoms. *Ment Health Phys Act*, Dec 2009; 2(2): 97–99.

58. Gomez-Pinilla F, Ying Z, Roy R et al. Voluntary exercise induces a BDNF–mediated mechanism that promotes neuroplasticity. *Journal of Neurophysiology*, 2002; 88(5): 2187–2195.

59. Erickson KI, Voss MW, Prakash RS. Exercise training increases size of hippocampus and improves memory. *PNAS*, 2011 Feb;108(7): 3017–3022.

60. Knaepen K, Goekint M, Heyman ME, Meeusen R. Neuroplasticity – exercise–induced response of peripheral brain–derived neurotropic factor. A systematic review of experimental studies in human subjects. *Sports Med*, Sept; 40(9): 765–801.

61. American Geriatric Society Panel on Exercise and Osteoarthritis. Exercise prescription for older adults with osteoarthritis pain: consensus practice recommendations. A supplement to the AGS Clinical Practice Guidelines on the management of chronic pain in older adults. *J Am Geriatr Soc*, 2001; 49(6): 808–23.

62. Haskell WL, Lee IM, Pate RR et al. Physical activity and public health: updated recommendation for adults from the American College of Sports Medicine and the American Heart Association. *Med Sci Sports Exerc*, 2007; 39 (8): 1423–34.

63. Lee IM, Sesso HD, Paffenbarger RS Jr. Physical activity and coronary heart disease risk in men: does the duration of the exercise episodes predict risk? *Circulation*, 2000; 102(9): 981–6.

64. Schoenfeld B, Dawes J. High–intensity interval training: applications for general fitness training. *Strength & Conditioning Journal*, Dec 2009; 31(6): 44–46.

65. Bouri, SZ, Arshadi S. Reaction of resting heart rate and blood pressure to high intensity interval and modern continuous training in coronary artery disease. *Br J Sports Med*, 2010; 44: i20.

66. Croft L, Bartlett JD, MacLaren DP et al. High-intensity interval training attenuates the exercise–induced increase in plasma IL-6 in response to acute exercise. *Appl Physiol Nutr Metab*, 2009; 34.

67. Garber CE, Blissmer B, Deschenes MR et al. Quantity and quality of exercise for developing and maintaining cardiorespiratory, musculoskeletal, and neuromotor fitness in apparently healthy adults: guidance for prescribing exercise. *Medicine & Science in Sports and Exercise*, 43(7):1334–59.

68. Jahnke R, Larkey L, Rogers C , Etnier J, Lin F. A comprehensive review of health benefits of Qigong and tai chi. *AM J Health Promot*, Jul–Aug 2010; 24 (6): c1-c25.

69. "Osteoporosis Exercise for Strong Bones." National Osteoporosis Foundation. https://www.nof.org/patients/treatment/exercisesafe-movement/osteoporosis-exercise-for-strong-bones/.

70. Clague J, Bernstein L. Physical activity and cancer. *Curr Oncol Rep*. 2012; 14(6):550–558.

71. Newton RU, Galvao DA. Exercise in prevention and management of cancer. *Curr Treat Options Oncol*. 2008; 9: 135–146.

72. Braga-Basaria M, Dobs AS, Muller DC et al. Metabolic syndrome in men with prostate cancer undergoing long-term androgen-deprivation therapy. *J Clin Oncol*, 2006; 2 (24): 3979–3983.

73. Zick C, et al. Harvesting More Than Vegetables: The Potential Weight Control Benefits of Community Gardening. *Am J Public Health*. 2013 June; 103(6): 1110–1115.

74. Dolgoff-Kaspar R, Baldwin A, Johnson MS. Effect of laughter yoga on mood and heart rate variability in patients awaiting organ transplantation: a pilot study. *Altern Ther Health Med*, 2012 Sep- Oct; 18(5): 61–6.

CHAPTER 15

1. Rothschild J, Hoddy KK, Jambazian P, Varady KA. Time-restricted feeding and risk of metabolic disease: a review of human and animal studies. *Nutr Rev.* 2014;72:308–18.

2. de Cabo R, Mattson MP. Effects of Intermittent Fasting on Health, Aging, and Disease. *NEJM*.2019; 381:2541–2551.

3. Moro T, Tinsley G, Bianco A, et al. Effects of eight weeks of time-restricted feeding (16/8) on basal metabolism, maximal strength, body composition, inflammation, and cardiovascular risk factors in resistance-trained males. *JTransl Med* 2016;14:290–290.4. Patterson RE, Laughlin GA, LaCroix AZ et al. Intermittent fasting and human metabolic health. *J Acad Nutr Diet.* 2015;115(8):1203–1212.

4. Hatori M, Vollmers C, Zarrinpar A et al. Time-restricted feeding without re-ducing caloric intake prevents metabolic diseases in mice fed a high-fat diet. *Cell Metab*.2012;15:848–860.

5. LeCheminant JD, Christenson E, Bailey BW et al. Restricting night time eat-ing reduces daily energy intake in healthy young men: a short-term cross-over study. *Br J Nutr*.2013;110 (11):2108–13.

6. Farooq N, Priyamvada S, Arivarasu NA et al. Influence of Ramadan-type fasting on enzymes of carbohydrate metabolism and brush border mem-brane in small intestine and liver of rat used a model. *Br J Nutr*. 2006;96: 1087–1094.

7. Temizhan A, Tandogan I, Docderici O et al. The effects of Ramadan fasting on blood lipid levels. *Am J Med*.2000;109:341–342.

8. Sherman H, Genzer Y, Cohen R et al. Timed high-fat diet resets circadian metabolism and prevents obesity. *FASEB J.* 2012;26 (8): 3493–502.

9. Ziaee V, Razaei M, Ahmadinejad Z et al. The changes of metabolic profile and weight during Ramadan fasting. *Singapore Med J.* 2006;47:409–414.

10. Sherman H, Frumin I, Gutman R et al. Long -term restricted feeding alters circadian expression and reduces the level of inflammatory and disease mark-ers. *J Cell Mol Med.* 2011;15:2745–2759.

11. Longo VD, Mattson MP. Fasting: molecular mechanisms and clinical appli-cations. *Cell Metab.* 2014;19(2):181–192.

12. Zarringpar A, Chaix A, Yooseph S, Panda S. Diet and Feeding Pattern Af-fect the Diurnal Dynamics of the Gut Microbiome. *Cell Metab.* 2014;20 (6):1006–1017.

13. Hayward S, Outlaw J, Urbina S et al. Effects of intermittent fasting on mark-ers of body composition and mood state. *Journal of International Sports Nutri-tion.* 2014; 11(Suppl 1):P25 http://www.jissn.com/content/11/S1/P25.

14. Witte AV, Fobker M, Gellner R et al. Caloric restriction improves memory in elderly humans. *Proc Natl Acad Sci USA* 2009;106:1255–1260.

15. Bachman JL, Deitrick RW, Hillman AR. Exercising in the Fasted State Reduced 24-Hour Energy Intake in Active Male Adults. *J Nutr Metab.* 2016; 2016:1984198.

16. Gonzalez JT, Veasey RC, Rumbold PLS, Stevenson EJ. Breakfast and exercise contingently affect postprandial metabolism and energy balance in physically active males. *British Journal of Nutrition.* 2013;110(4):721–732.

CHAPTER 16

1. Rasmussen HN, Scheirer M, Greenhouse JB. Optimism and Physical Health: A Meta-analytic Review. *Ann Behav Med.* 2009; 37(3):239–256.

2. Conversano C, Rotondo A, Lensi E et al. Optimism and Its Impact on Mental and Physical Well- Being. *Clin Pract Epidemiol Mental Health.* 2010; 6:25–29.

3. Rozanski A, Bavishi C, Kubzansky et al. Association of Optimism with Cardiovascular Events and All-Cause Mortality. A Systematic Review and Meta-analysis. *JAMA Netw Open.* 2019; 2 (9): e191220.

4. Scheier MF, Carver CS. Optimism, coping, and health assessment and implications of generalized outcome expancies. *Health Psychol.* 1985;4(3) 21–47.

5. Lee L, James P, Zevon E et al. Optimism is associated with exceptional longevity in 2 epidemiologic cohorts of men and women. *PNAS,* 2019 Sep 10; 116(37):18357–18362.

6. Sharot T, Guitart-Masip M, Korn CW et al. How dopamine enhances an optimism bias in humans. *Curr Biol.* 2012 Aug 21;22(16):1477–81.

7. Seligman, Martin. *Flourish.* New York, NY. Free Press, 2011

8. Achor, Shawn. *The Happiness Advantage.* New York, NY. Ebury Publishing, 2010.

9. Howren MB, Lamkin DM, Suls J. Association of depression with C-reactive protein, IL-1, and Il-6: a meta-analysis. *Psychosom Med.* 2009; 47:142–147.

10. Dowlati Y, Herrmann N, Swardfager W et al. A meta-analysis of cytokines in major depression. *Biol. Psychiatry.* 2010; 446–457.

11. Pariante CM, Lightman SL. The HPA axis in major depression: classical theories and new developments. *Trends Neuroscience.* 2008;31:464–468.

GLOSSARY

Acanthosis nigricans: Black or brown discoloration of the skin that is found in skin folds, such as the armpits, neck, and groin.

Adenosine: A neurotransmitter in the brain that can promote sleep and suppress arousal.

ADHD: Attention deficit hyperactivity disorder; a medical condition characterized by difficulty staying focused, paying attention, controlling behavior, and hyperactivity.

Adiponectin: A hormone produced and secreted by fat cells that regulate metabolism of glucose and fats.

Adrenaline: Also known as epinephrine; a neurotransmitter that is released by the adrenal gland in response to stress.

Aerobic: Exercise that is intended to improve the efficiency of the cardiovascular system in absorbing and transporting oxygen.

Alpha-linolenic acid (ALA): A fatty acid that is essential for health and cannot be made by the body, so it must be consumed through diet; a precursor to the formation of omega-3 fatty acids.

Alzheimer's disease: A form of memory loss that is the most common form of dementia; characterized by amyloid plaques.

American Academy of Environmental Medicine: An international organization that represents physicians who specialize in looking at the interactions of environment and its impact on health.

Amino acids: Building blocks of protein.

Anabolic hormones: Hormones that are primarily in charge of building the body.

Anaerobic: During exercise, when oxygen demands cannot be kept up and the formation of lactic acid is triggered.

Antioxidants: Substances that may prevent or delay types of cell damage.

Asanas: Physical aspect of yoga that relates to benefits from the postures.

Atherosclerosis: The buildup of plaque in and on artery walls.

Atherosclerotic plaque: Plaque in the blood vessel (artery) walls.

ATP: Adenosine triphosphate; the end product in many cellular reactions that serves as an energy source.

Atrophy: A tissue or organ that wastes away due to degeneration of the cells.

Auditory learning: The act of learning new material through sound and speech.

Autism: An illness characterized by difficulties in social interactions and verbal and nonverbal communication, and is notable for repetitive behavior.

Autoimmune disease: A class of illness that involves the overactivation of the immune system, forcing the body to attack its own tissues.

Autonomic nervous system: A part of the nervous system that influences the function of internal organs.

Beta brain waves: EEG patterns found to represent activity of the brain when it is alert, engaged in problem-solving, focused on activity, or making judgments or decisions.

Body composition: A calculation of the percentage of fat, muscle, bone, and water in a human.

Body mass index (BMI): Height-to-weight ratio that categorizes people as normal size, overweight, and obese; obesity is associated with development of chronic disease.

Brain-derived neurotrophic factor (BDNF): A protein that has a role in supporting survival of existing neurons and is vital to learning and memory.

Calorie: One calorie is the energy required to raise the temperature of one gram of water by one degree.

Calorie density: Calories per amount of food; high calorie-dense foods have more calories by weight or volume than low caloric-dense foods.

Carbohydrates: A type of nutrient found in food that is important for energy production and forms into glucose.

Carcinogens: Any substance or compound that can be directly involved with causing cancer.

Cardiac catheterization: A procedure in which a small tube is placed in a blood vessel; dye placed in the catheter helps visualize blockages in the vessels surrounding the heart.

Cardiac C-reactive protein: More specific measure of inflammation in the heart.

Cardiovascular disease/heart disease: Class of illness that involves the heart and blood vessels.

Cardiovascular system: A system in the body that involves the heart and blood vessels.

Carotenoids: Yellow, orange, or red pigments found in plants, such as fruits and vegetables, that offer antioxidant benefits to cells.

Casein: The protein found in milk and dairy products.

Celiac disease: A genetically predisposing autoimmune disease characterized by damage to the lining of the small intestine due to a severe reaction to gluten.

Cerebrospinal fluid: Clear fluid found in the brain and the spine that acts as a protective cushion for the brain and spinal cord.

Chromosomes: Structures inside the nucleus of a cell that house the DNA.

Circadian rhythm: A cycle of 24 hours that can affect physical, mental, and behavioral changes.

Cognition: The process of acquiring knowledge through thought.

Collagen: The structural protein in the space outside cells that offers strength and structure to our bodies.

Clostridium difficile colitis (C. diff): An inflammatory illness of the large intestine secondary to a bacteria called Clostridium difficile.

Colon cancer: A type of cancer that affects the large intestine or rectum.

Colorectal cancer: Often an umbrella term used for cancer of the colon.

Constipation: A condition where there is difficulty emptying the bowels often due to dehydration; associated with hardened stools.

COPD: Chronic obstructive pulmonary disease; a medical illness characterized by blocked airflow and difficulty breathing.

Coronary arteries: The blood vessels that supply the heart muscle.

Coronary calcium score: A measure of plaque levels in blood vessels.

Cortisol: A hormone secreted by the adrenal gland that is released in response to stress.

C-reactive protein: A blood test that is used to gauge and monitor inflammation; nonspecific and could suggest inflammation anywhere in the body.

Cytokines: Small proteins involved with cell signaling.

Dementia: A general term that implies a decline in mental function that is severe enough to impact daily life.

Detoxification: Removal of substances that can be poisonous to our body.

DHEA: A hormone secreted by the adrenal gland.

Diabetes: An illness that is categorized by difficulty processing glucose; different types of diabetes are based on whether insulin is being generated by the pancreas; diagnosis is made if fasting glucose level measures over 126 twice or more or if the HBA1c is over 6.5 g/dL.

Distress: The detrimental effects of stress to the mind and body.

Diverticulosis: A medical condition characterized by the presence of small pouches in the large intestine.

Dysbiosis: A condition where the bacterial flora is not in balance.

E. coli: Gram negative bacteria that is part of normal gut flora.

Elementary prevention: Tools that we use to prevent the onset of illness.

Endocrine: A system in the body that produces hormones that regulate many functions of the body, such as metabolism, growth and development, reproduction, sexual function, sleep, and mood.

Endometrial: Pertaining to the lining of the uterus.

Endorphins: Naturally produced by the brain; these peptides have opiate-like activities and can reduce pain naturally.

Endothelium: Single cell layer that lines the interior surface of the blood vessels.

Epinephrine: A hormone released by the adrenal gland during a stress response that raises the heart rate and blood pressure.

Essential fatty acids: Fats that cannot be generated from the body and must be taken in through the diet; examples are linoleic and alpha-linolenic acid.

Eustress: A term coined by Hans Seyle, MD; the beneficial effects of stress on the mind and body.

Fermentation: Metabolic process that involves the conversion of sugar to gases, alcohol, or acids.

Firmicutes: Bacteria found in the gut.

Flavonoid: A plant-based compound found in fruits and vegetables that offers antioxidant benefits; common foods high in flavonoids are onions, parsley, blueberries, bananas, dark chocolate, and red wine.

Free radicals: Harmful toxins triggered by stress.

Fructose: A simple sugar that combines with glucose to form sucrose.

Functional medicine: Type of medicine that focuses on a multisystem approach to disease; focuses on the interactions of the environment and the gastrointestinal, endocrine, and immune systems.

Galactose: The sugar found in milk and dairy products.

General adaptation syndrome: The physiologic process of how the body responds to a new stress.

Genes: Basic unit of heredity; made up of DNA; they make us who we are.

Genetically modified (GMO): A food or crop that has genetic material that has been artificially altered.

Genome: Complete set of DNA of an organism.

Germ-free host: Usually a rat or mouse that has had of all of its microbiota eradicated.

Ghrelin: A hormone that has a role in triggering appetite.

Glucose: An umbrella term for sugar; used as energy for our cells; high levels are associated with diabetes.

Glutathione: An antioxidant made naturally in the liver.

Glycemic index: Numerical index from zero to 100 that ranks carbohydrates by the rate of their conversion to glucose in the body; a food with a higher glycemic index rating converts more easily to glucose.

Glycogenolysis: The breakdown of glycogen into glucose.

Gut-brain axis: The connection that is based on the biochemical signaling between the nervous system (brain) and the gastrointestinal tract (gut).

HDL: A type of cholesterol that is favorable to health.

Heterocyclic amines: Compounds that are created when cooking foods at high temperature.

Hippocampus: A part of the brain that has a major role in memory.

HIV: Human immunodeficiency virus; causes marked suppression of the immune system.

Homeostasis: The tendency of the body to create internal stability and equilibrium, despite stressors; the body's need to have balance.

Hormones: Proteins in the blood that travel from one site to another to cause changes.

Hydrogenated oil: Where a hydrogen bond is added to liquid oil to turn it into a solid; increases shelf life of a product.

Hygiene hypothesis: A theory that states that a decreased early exposure to infectious agents, good microorganisms, and parasites increases risk to allergenic disease by suppressing the natural development of our immune system.

Hypertension: An illness in which a person has persistently elevated blood pressure.

Hypertrophy: Enlargement of a tissue or organ.

IL-6: Cytokine that has a strong role in stimulating an inflammatory response during infections and trauma.

Immune system: The system in the body that works to protect the body from disease; a system that fights against infections and other abnormal cells.

Inflammation: The presence of an activated immune system that produces chemicals when there are injuries, infection, damaged cells, or irritants in the body.

Inflammatory bowel disease: Chronic inflammation of part or all of the digestive tract; can be associated with abdominal pain, bloody diarrhea, and joint pain.

Insomnia: The symptom of the inability to sleep.

Insulin: A hormone required for the cells to take up glucose .

Insulin resistance (IR): A condition where the cells of the body become increasingly resistant to the effects of insulin.

Interstitial space: The space between cells of a tissue that are fluid filled.

Intestinal permeability: Weakening of the bowel wall.

Irritable bowel syndrome: A chronic intestinal disorder with symptoms such as as cramping, bloating, constipation, and diarrhea.

Isometric: Type of strength training in which the joint angle does not change, such as with planks.

Isotonic: A type of exercise where the joint angle and muscle length change and muscle tone is kept constant during movement; examples are squats, push-ups, and pull-ups.

Ketosis: A metabolic process where there is low availability of carbohydrates, and energy production has to come primarily from fat sources.

Kilocalorie: Used frequently to identify the energy obtained by intake of food; 1,000 calories equal one kilocalorie; often used interchangeably with calorie.

Lactic acid: Normal by-product of anaerobic muscle metabolism that is associated with discomfort and soreness.

Lactose: Sugar made from galactose and glucose and primarily found in milk and dairy products.

LDL: A type of cholesterol that is implicated in forming plaque.

Leptin: A hormone made by fat cells that regulates hunger and helps us feel full.

Lignans: Chemical compounds found in plants; have antioxidant effects.

Linoleic acid (LA): A fatty acid that is essential for health and cannot be made by the body, so it must be consumed through the diet; part of the omega-6– fatty acid chain.

Lipolysis: The breakdown of fats and lipids.

Lipopolysaccharide: Molecules found on the outer membrane of certain types of bacteria that can elicit a strong immune response.

Lupus: Short for systemic lupus erythematosus, an autoimmune disease that can affect skin, joints, and organs in the body.

Macrophages: White cells of the immune system that are associated with defense against infection by foreign cells, eliminating damaged cells, and the formation of plaque.

Macular degeneration: An illness associated with damage to the retina of the eye; can cause blindness and visual impairment in adults.

Malabsorption: Characterized by a difficulty in absorption of nutrients from food.

Mammillary bodies: Part of the brain that is involved in recognition memory, such as remembering that you had seen someone before.

Maximum predicted heart rate (MPHR): A measure calculated by subtracting someone's age from 220; achieving 85 percent MPHR is associated with better cardiovascular outcomes.

Melatonin: A hormone that promotes sleep.

Metabolic equivalent of tasks (MET): A physiologic measure that expresses the energy cost of physical activities.

Metabolic fitness: The benefits that occur when muscles become more efficient at utilizing their resources; indirectly can be measured by glucose tolerance and lipid profiles.

Metabolism: Process by which there is conversion of food into energy; often referred to in terms of weight management.

Microbiome: The collective genome of the microorganisms that share our body.

Microbiota: The collective community of microorganisms that share our body.

Microorganisms: A living organism that is single celled and is microscopic.

Mindfulness: A meditative state where the focus of attention is on the present moment.

Mitochondria: A vital part of cells and tissues where energy production occurs.

Monounsaturated fats: A fatty acid or fat where there is one double bond, often found in olive oil.

Multiple sclerosis: An autoimmune illness where the immune system attacks the protective covering of nerves.

Myelin sheaths: The protective covering of nerves, including the brain and spinal cord; allows electrical impulses to transmit efficiently along nerves.

Myocardial infarction: Plaque rupture in the heart that causes damage to the heart muscle by restricting blood supply.

National Sleep Foundation: An organization that has resources for sleep research and education regarding sleep disorders.

Natural killer cells: Type of white cells that respond to viral infections and tumor cells.

Nerve conduction: The movement of an electrical impulse along a nerve.

Neurocognitive disorder: An illness that causes progressive deterioration of the nervous system, leading to deterioration of the ability to formulate new knowledge and access and process existing knowledge.

Neurodegenerative conditions: A broad term for illnesses that primarily affect the neurons in the brain.

Neuroplasticity: The ability of neural pathways to change due to changes in behavior, environment, thinking, emotions, injury, and disease.

Neuroprotective: Something that has the ability to protect the brain, spinal cord, and nerves.

Neurotoxins: Any chemical or substance that can cause damage to a nerve cell.

Neurotransmitters: Chemicals that transmit signals across nerve cells.

Nitric oxide (NO): A gas that dilates the blood vessels.

Nonsense syllables: Syllables that have no meaning; used in songs, memory experiments, or tests.

Norepinephrine: A hormone released by the adrenal gland during a stress response that raises the heart rate and blood pressure.

Obesity: A term used to define excess weight; defined by a BMI of 30 kg/m2 or higher.

Omega-3 fatty acids: Polyunsaturated fats that are broken down into eicosapentaenoic acids (EPA) and docosahexaenoic acids (DHA); found in walnuts, chia seeds, and flax seeds.

Osteoarthritis: A type of degenerative arthritis mostly due to wear and tear.

Overreaching syndrome: A compilation of symptoms that occurs when the balance between training and recovery is not proportionate; usually lasts two weeks.

Overtraining: Training that is significantly outweighed by recovery; causes a compilation of symptoms that can last weeks to months.

Overweight: A term used to define excess weight; defined by a BMI between 25 and 29.9 kg/m2.

Oxidative stress: Stress on the body that triggers formation of toxic chemicals, free radicals.

Pancreatic cancer: A type of cancer that affects the pancreas.

Parasympathetic nervous system: One division of the autonomic nervous system that regulates the body's rest-and-digestive system in times of calm and relaxation.

Parkinson's disease: A medical illness that is characterized by a movement disorder associated with a resting tremor.

Pasteurization: A process of heating that is intended to reduce the number of microorganisms in foods.

Percentage body fat: The amount of fat in our bodies.

Phosphatidylcholine: A lipid found on the membrane of cells.

Photosensitive retinal ganglion cells: A type of nerve cell in the retina of the eye that signals the presence of light.

Phytoestrogens: Plant-derived natural substances that have structural similarity to estrogen made by the ovaries; can bind to estrogen receptors and can cause estrogenic or antiestrogenic effects.

Phytonutrients: Chemicals in plants, such as fruits and vegetables, that protect them from environmental and infectious agents; also have health-promoting properties, such as high contents of antioxidants and other anti-inflammatory substances.

Pineal gland: A small endocrine gland in the brain that secretes melatonin.

Plant sterols: Naturally occurring substances found in grains, vegetables, fruits, legumes, nuts, and seeds that have cholesterol-lowering properties.

Plaque: A substance made up of fat, cholesterol, calcium, and inflammatory cells found in the blood; can harden and block flow of oxygen-rich blood over time.

Platelet aggregation: The act of the platelet cells sticking together to help stop bleeding and form a clot.

Polycyclic aromatic hydrocarbons: Organic compounds that are formed when there is insufficient oxygen; often found when foods are cooked at high temperatures and thought to be carcinogenic.

Polycystic ovary syndrome: A medical condition characterized by the presence of insulin resistance associated with menstrual irregularities, infertility, abnormal glucose, and excessive hair growth in women.

Polyunsaturated fats: A fatty acid or fat where there is more than one double bond; found in many vegetable oils.

Positron emission tomography: Type of imaging test using radioactive dye that allows us to detect disease in the body.

Pranayama breathing: Formal practice of control and extension of breath.

Prediabetes: Mild elevations in blood glucose.

Prefrontal cortex: An area of the brain in the frontal lobe that is implicated in planning complex cognitive behavior, personality expression, and decision-making.

Preservative: A substance that is added to food and beverages to help prevent its decomposition by the growth of microbes or by chemical changes.

Probiotics: Ingested microorganisms that replenish gut flora.

Protein: Large molecules that are composed of amino acids.

Psychomotor performance: Coordination of motor activity with a sensory or cognitive process.

Receptors: A region on a cell membrane that responds to a particular hormone or substance.

REM sleep: A stage of sleep characterized by rapid eye movements; considered the dream state.

Resistance exercise: Exercise that causes a muscle to contract against external resistance.

Resistant starches: Type of dietary fiber naturally found in carbohydrate foods that can help grow the good bacteria in our digestive tract.

Resveratrol: A natural chemical produced in plants in response to an injury or when the plant is under attack by a fungus or bacteria; found in high levels in the skin of grapes.

Rheumatoid arthritis: An autoimmune illness where the immune system attacks the joints.

Saponins: Chemical compounds found in plants that are thought to protect the plant against microbes and fungi.

Saturated fat: A type of fat that has no double bonds; found in animal fats and many oils.

Serotonin: A biochemical regulator or neurotransmitter that is thought to regulate mood; predominantly found in the GI tract.

Short-chain fatty acids: End products of fermentation of fiber by anaerobic bacteria of the intestinal lining that have shown to exert multiple beneficial effects.

Sivasana: A pose in yoga for total relaxation; also called the corpse pose.

Sleep apnea: A medical condition characterized by disruption of sleep due to low oxygen levels in the brain.

Sleep fragmentation: The disturbance in sleep that is notable for interruption of the sleep stages.

Sleep latency: The amount of time it takes from lying down to sleep until the onset of sleep.

Statins: Medications to lower cholesterol.

Stroke: An illness where poor blood flow to the brain causes injury and even the death of brain cells.

Stroke volume: The amount of blood pumped out of the heart with each contraction.

Subconscious: Part of the mind that is not fully aware but can influence actions and feelings.

Subcutaneous fat: The fat under the skin.

Sympathetic nervous system: One division of the autonomic nervous system that regulates the body's fight-or-flight response in times of stress and danger.

Sympathetic overdrive: The state of having a persistent activation to a stress response.

T cell: A type of white blood cell that is part of the immune system; responsible for fighting infection.

Telomeres: The region at the ends of a chromosome that protects it from deterioration.

TMAO: Trimethylamine N-oxide; a substance formed by bacteria in the gut which promotes the formation of plaque in our blood vessels.

TNF (TNF-alpha): Tumor necrosis factor, a cell-signaling protein released by the immune system in response to insult and involved in acute phase reaction; recruits cells that invoke a response to stress, inflammation, and infections.

Toxins: Substances that can be poisonous to our body.

Trans fats: Chemically engineered fats that are used to make oils more solid at room temperature; increases shelf life.

Triglycerides: A type of fat that is found in the blood; high levels are thought to be a risk factor for heart disease.

Tryptophan: An amino acid that is a precursor to serotonin; considered an essential amino acid since your body cannot make it; must be consumed.

Type 1 diabetes: A disorder of glucose metabolism resulting from an auto-immune process where the body attacks the insulin-forming cells and the pancreas cannot generate insulin.

Type 2 diabetes: High blood sugar levels due to the resistance of the body to the actions of insulin.

Unsaturated fats: A fatty acid or fat where there are one or more double bonds, found in vegetable oils, avocados, and nuts.

Vagus nerve: A nerve that spreads into the gastrointestinal tract and the heart and is a large component of the parasympathetic nervous system.

Visceral fat: Fat that surrounds organs in the abdominal cavity.

World Health Organization: Health arm of the United Nations that focuses on international public health.

Yoga nidra: A form of guided meditation that helps with relaxation.

ACKNOWLEDGMENTS

We would like to acknowledge a few people without whom this book would not have been possible. First, we want to thank Dr. Parthiv Mahadevia and ERS, who have helped read and reread and reread the chapters of the book. We would also like to thank Mona Shroff and Kosha Dalal for helping with edits and Anjali Shroff for helping us by taking great food photos. We would like to thank Shilpa Johnson for giving us innovative recipes. We would like to thank Philip Hicks, who helped us personally to get stronger and helped us put together exercises for all ages. We also would like to thank two very influential people: Karen Fick is an amazing person and helped Dr. Aggarwal start on her journey to healing. Dr. A will always be thankful to her for that. We also want to thank Bob Lascaro who has been an amazing designer, advisor, and guide with putting this book together and without whom, none of this would have been possible. Dr. R says thank you to her kids, Anjali, Shalin, and Kiren, for supporting her through this journey. Last but not least, thank you to Bob and Cynthia Holzapfel for helping us take this book to the next level.

MONICA AGGARWAL graduated from the University of Virginia in 1996 with a major in religious studies and a minor in biology and from the Medical College of Virginia in Richmond, Virginia, in 2000 with a degree in medicine. She did her internal medicine residency at Tufts University Hospital from 2000 until 2003. Subsequently, she went on to do her cardiology fellowship at the University of Maryland in Baltimore from 2003 until 2006. She also did an integrative medicine fellowship at the University of Arizona Integrative Medicine center. She is board certified in cardiology, echocardiography, and nuclear cardiology.

Dr. Aggarwal is now clinical associate professor of medicine at the University of Florida Division of Cardiovascular Medicine, where she also serves as the director of integrative cardiology and prevention. In her clinic, she emphasizes plant-based nutrition and often performs multiple mind-body techniques with her patients, including yoga and meditation. She has instituted a new nationally acclaimed plant-based menu at the Shands Hospital of the University of Florida, along with new discharge education that empowers patients to heal their bodies with their lifestyles. She was recently named Florida's "Cardiovascular Researcher of the Year" by the Florida chapter of the American College of Cardiology, which provided her with a grant to conduct important research needed on nutrition. She speaks nationally on deficits in nutrition education and how to implement healthy lifestyle into clinical practice.

JYOTHI RAO graduated from Rutgers University in 1990 with a major in biology and from New Jersey Medical School in Newark, New Jersey, in 1994 with a degree in medicine. She did her internal medicine residency at Tufts-New England Medical Center from 1994 until 1997. She has worked in clinical practice since 1997. She completed her medical acupuncture training at the Helms Institute of Acupuncture in UCLA in 2000. She completed her fellowship in functional medicine from the American Academy of Anti-Aging and Regenerative Medicine in 2013. She is also an instructor at the Maryland University of Integrative Health. She is currently the medical director of the Shakthi Health and Wellness Center. She is board certified in internal medicine and antiaging and regenerative medicine.

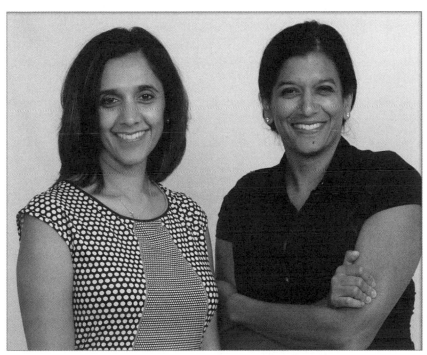

Jyothi Rao (left) and Monica Aggarwal (right)

INDEX

Page references for sidebars are *italicized*.

A

acanthosis nigricans, 32, 221
Achor, Shawn, 191
adenosine triphosphate (ATP)/adenosine, 122, 126, 145, 165, 166, 221
ADHD (attention deficit hyperactivity disorder), 121, 221
adiponectin, 146, 221
adrenaline, 126, *127, 137,* 145, 147, 167, 221
aerobic exercise/metabolism, 221
   anaerobic exercise/metabolism vs., 165–66, *166,* 169–71, *170*
   calories burned and, *165*
   cardiovascular (coronary artery/heart) disease and, 173
   cognition and, 177
   fat burning and, 166, 170
   lifestyle and, 84
   METs and, 161, *162*
   varied workouts and, 172, *184*
   weight loss and, 164
aging
   attitude about, 11
   cognition and, 20, 177–78
   cortisol and, 19
   exercise and, 178, 179
   hormones and, 146
   ketones and, 186
   meditation and, 145–46
   mindfulness and, 145
   phytonutrients and, 74
   sleep and, 124
   stress and, 144
   telomeres and, 19–20
   yoga and, 143, *144,* 144–46

alignment/posture exercises, *182–83*
allergies, 4, 37, 42–43, 49–50, 58
alpha-linolenic acid (ALA), 78, 85, 94, *94,* 104–5, 106, 221
Alzheimer's disease, 221
   coconut oil and, 101
   death (mortality) and, 24
   gut bacteria (flora) and, 48
   ketones and, 186
   LPS and, 41
   meditation and, 149
   turmeric and, 112
amino acids, 221
   arginine/L-arginine, 102, 103–4
   exercise and, 168, *169*
   gut and, 37
   protein and, 229
   as resource, 2
   in specific foods, 60, 115, 168, *169*
   tryptophan/L-tryptophan, 47, 48, 105, 231
anabolic hormones, 173, 221
anaerobic exercise/metabolism, 165, 166, *166, 170,* 170–71, 221, 226, 230
animal foods/products. *See also* specific types of
   in Africans'/African-American diets, 38
   eliminating from diet, 55–58
   GMOs and, 70, 71
   as inflammation source, 8
   leaky gut and, 49
   in patient cases, 53, 54
   protein and, 65
   saturated fats and, 91, 93, 230
   as unhealthful, 63, 71, 87, 106
antioxidants, 187, 221. *See also* specific types of

arthritis, x, 32, 110, 111–12, *112,* 140. *See also* specific types of
artificial colorings and/or flavorings, 66, 70
artificial sweeteners, 67–69, *68, 69,* 70, 72
asanas, *141,* 142, 148, 152, 221
atherosclerosis/atherosclerotic plaque, 221
   coconut oil and, 101
   endothelial dysfunction and, 27
   high cholesterol and, 30
   lifestyle and, 84
   saturated fats and, 92, 98–99
   turmeric and, 113
atrophy, 149, 221
auditory learning, 149, 221
autism, 41, 48, 222
autoimmune disease(s), 222. *See also* specific diseases
   body imbalance and, x
   childhood nutrition and, 30
   cortisol and, 19
   gut bacteria/microbiome and, 37, 43–44
   increase in, 3, 24, 50
   milk and, 63
   treatment for, 49
autonomic nervous system, 15, *16,* 46, 126, 154, 222, 228, 230
autophagy, 187, 188
avocados, 100–101, 106, *107*

B

beans
   amino acids and, 168, *169*
   butyrate production and, 88
   calcium in, 8, 60
   canned, 67, *67*
   carbohydrates and, 79–80
   as healthful, 88, *89*

234

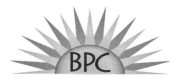

books that educate, inspire, and empower

To find your favorite books on plant-based cooking and nutrition,
raw-foods cuisine, and healthy living, visit:
BookPubCo.com

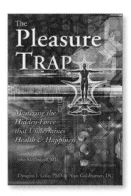

The Pleasure Trap
Douglas J. Lisle, PhD
Alan Goldhamer, DC
978-1-57067-197-5 • $14.95

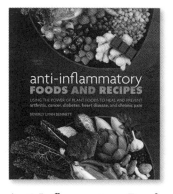

*Anti-Inflammatory Foods
and Recipes*
Beverly Lynn Bennett
978-1-57067-341-2 • $17.95

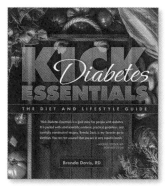

Kick Diabetes Essentials
Brenda Davis, RD
978-1-57067-376-4 • $24.95

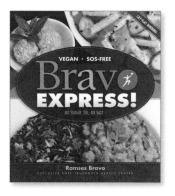

Bravo Express!
Ramses Bravo
978-1-57067-362-7 • $22.95

Purchase these titles from your favorite book source or buy them directly from:
Book Publishing Company • PO Box 99 • Summertown, TN 38483 • 1-888-260-8458
Free shipping and handling on all orders